P9-ARE-798

PRAISE FOR

DIET FOR DIVINE CONNECTION

"I have loved Margaret Paul's teachings for over twenty years. She has always been ahead of her time and continues to be a renegade leading thinker and teacher in the psycho-emotional and spiritual realm with this book. Margaret deftly combines profound and integrated teachings for our modern times with certainty, experience, and great clarity ... all the while living what she teaches.

"Her holistic way of looking at well-being is inspirational, leading edge, and a great gift to anyone wanting support emotionally, physically, spiritually, and mentally.

"This new book finds her evolving and integrating even more of her learned and hard-won wisdom by including even more aspects of our humanness ... our bodies, our food choices, and our minds and brains, all the while continuing to point us home to our true and most sacred selves. I am so happy Margaret Paul is on this Earth."

— Alanis Morissette, singer, songwriter, teacher, and visionary

"Dr. Margaret Paul spent years uncovering the ways we can connect with our guidance and how that is related to the many different kinds of nourishment (both physical and emotional) we give our bodies. In *Diet For Divine Connection*, you will discover how to heal resistance to physical and emotional self-care and how to lovingly act on your own behalf in any moment. Margaret Paul is connected with her own internal GPS. [She] teaches us how to do the same, and in the process, so much healing takes place. We're fortunate to have her as our guide."

— Geneen Roth, author of *This Messy Magnificent Life* and the #1 New York Times best-selling book *Women Food and God*

"In her magnificent new work, *Diet for Divine Connection*, Dr. Margaret Paul has given us deep and immediate access to the unshakable foundations of inner security, vitality, and a high-frequency consciousness. Only with these foundations can we experience the happiness and authentic success we desire and deserve in our lives. She shares not only from her vast expertise and decades of work, research, and practice but from the source of wisdom itself, which can only be accessed by someone who has embodied and lived all she offers to others. Her book is a rare and potent transmission that will heal, integrate, and ignite your mind, body, heart, and soul into wholeness."

— Claire Zammit, PhD, founder of *FemininePower.com*

"This wonderful book will help you align your mind-body-spirit to create a healthy, vibrant, life-affirming diet. Food is medicine. Food is spirit. Dr. Margaret Paul is a skilled, empathic teacher and beautiful human being. In this book, she lovingly shows you how to access your Divine guidance and how listening to your Divine guidance will support you to choose the right foods for your body and restore your wholeness and well-being."

— Judith Orloff MD, author of *The Empath's Survival Guide*

"Junk food and junk thoughts both have the same net effect. They clog you up and limit your vitality and your capacity for joy. In this penetrating and provocative book, Dr. Paul illumines how it's all connected and invites you on a pathway to greater mental, physical, and spiritual wellness."

— Ocean Robbins, CEO of Food Revolution Network

"According to the reports from thousands of individuals and numerous physicians, when people switch to a non-GMO organic diet, they experience dramatic improvements in health, clarity, concentration, weight loss, memory, and energy. Many recover from anxiety and depression. The toxins in food have robbed millions of their health and vitality. Reversing this trend sets the stage for the kind of life we all desire. Healthy food is the urgent first step. Thank you, Margaret, for ringing that bell."

— Jeffrey M. Smith, founder of the Institute for Responsible Technology and best-selling author and filmmaker

"Margaret Paul has synthesized a remarkable amount of research, sharing a wealth of insights on what and how we eat and think are connected to our physical, mental, emotional states as well as our spiritual consciousness and ability to evolve. She brilliantly shares with us how we can raise our frequency, giving us deeper access to our ability to connect with the Divine.

"After absorbing life-changing information, readers are masterfully led into Margaret Paul's powerful Inner Bonding work. Through experiential exercises and case studies, readers are taught life-changing skills to heal what is disconnecting them from their divine selves.

"*Diet for Divine Connection* is truly remarkable, filled with so many resources. I will use this book as a guide to read again and again. This book is a true gift and speaks well to how to navigate the times we are living in."

— Sandra Ingerman, MA, author twelve books, including *Soul Retrieval* and *Walking in Light*

"Profound and practical insights for integrating the psychology of healing our hearts with the foods we eat to expand our consciousness and strengthen our divine connection with spirit."

— John Gray, PhD, best-selling author of *Men Are From Mars, Women Are From Venus*

"*Diet For Divine Connection* is a wise, comprehensive, integral guide to good health on all levels. In it, the masterful Margaret Paul offers us an in-depth and accessible roadmap to learn how to love ourselves through aligning our thoughts, actions, and food choices with great wisdom and love. A magically transformative book for all serious seekers of health, healing and wholeness. I highly recommend it!"

— Katherine Woodward Thomas, New York Times best-selling author of *Calling in "The One"* and *Conscious Uncoupling*

"I believe the best testimonial for this brilliant book is Dr. Margaret Paul herself! I have known Dr. Paul for more than thirty-four years, and I can tell you without hesitation that her youthful vitality, energy, and health are extraordinary. She has researched and lived the information contained in these pages for more than fifty years, and it is clear to me that this woman *knows* something! We can all benefit from the wisdom and research contained in these pages. Dr. Paul maintains a crushing schedule with ease and then still has energy to gallop her horse across the fields or take her kayak out fishing or spend hours in her art studio! Dr. Paul is seventy-eight years old! If there is a fountain of health framed in academia, it is here in these pages. I invite you to partake in her wisdom and live your life to its fullest like Dr. Margaret Paul."

— Erika J. Chopich, PhD, co-author of *Healing Your Aloneness* and *The Healing Your Aloneness Workbook* and cocreator of Inner Bonding and SelfQuest

"*Diet for Divine Connection* cuts through the conflicting theories on nutrition, empowering the reader to make intelligent food choices for optimal well-being on every level. It addresses the psychological reasons that often hold a person back from implementing positive changes, which come down to a lack of self-love. Most remarkable is Margaret Paul's understanding of the spiritual impact of our food diet and thought diet. With great wisdom and compassion, she shows us how we can embody an inspired, graceful, vital existence, even in these challenging times. This is truly a groundbreaking contribution. Read it and reap!"

— Miranda Macpherson, author of *Boundless Love* and *The Way of Grace: the Transforming Power of Ego Relaxation* (October, 2018)

"In this breakthrough work, Dr. Margaret Paul brings us the science that connects diet and the Divine. Dr. Paul also teaches us how to overcome any blocks to loving ourselves so that we can let go of junk foods and junk thoughts and open to at-will Divine connection. Read it — it will forever change your understanding of food and spirituality, and how to embrace the thought and action choices necessary to achieve Divine connection."

— Hyla Cass MD, author of *8 Weeks to Vibrant Health*

"*Diet for Divine Connection* may be the most useful and healing book about diet and nutrition I've ever read. Margaret Paul explains that the only truly effective diet is one that springs from your own inner guidance and intuition. In clear and simple terms, Dr. Paul teaches you exactly how to use your intuition to create both a food and a thought diet that heals and enlivens your entire being. No matter your age, health, or dietary challenges, *Diet for Divine Connection* can save you years of struggle. Best of all, because it's truly a soul-based path to physical and emotional health, you'll discover life-changing new inner reservoirs of energy, peace, and precious clarity. If you care about your health and well-being, don't miss this treasure of a book.

— Ken Page, LCSW, author of *Deeper Dating: How to Drop the Games of Seduction and Discover the Power of Intimacy*

"This is not just another book about food and the body. It weaves together many other aspects of a healthy life: the importance of high-vibration foods that resonate with your essence, the power of your 'state' when you eat and digest, and the full presence of you-the-soul to guide self-nurturing. This is a valuable and comprehensive guidebook for transforming your entire self at the physical, emotional, mental, and spiritual levels."

— Penney Peirce, author of *Transparency, Frequency,* and *Leap of Perception*

"A powerful message whose time has come! Dr. Margaret Paul's *Diet for Divine Connection* is a cutting-edge spiritual look at how junk food and 'junk thoughts' sabotage our connection to the Divine. Margaret's proven processes will support you in shedding old habits and false beliefs so that you can live, love, and lead from your inner wisdom and create a life of radiant health and inner peace."

— Linda Joy, visibility catalyst, best-selling publisher, and publisher of *Aspire Magazine,* www.Linda-Joy.com

"If you're ready to discover the root causes of disconnection from self, others, and Divine guidance, then *Diet For Divine Connection* is a must-read, groundbreaking book. For anyone desiring mind, body, and spirit healing, Dr. Paul clearly describes the connection between the foods you eat and the thoughts you think with your ability to connect with your Divine guidance — your inner GPS — and she offers a pathway to healing through her six-step Inner Bonding process."

— Charlotte Reznick, PhD, author of *The Power of Your Child's Imagination: How to Transform Stress and Anxiety into Joy and Success*

"This book will change lives! Dr. Margaret Paul has connected the dots no one else has, bringing together the relationship between the food we eat, the thoughts we think, and our inner awareness of our Divine self. These are all interdependent aspects of our humanity, and this book explains how to make the connections in order to live a vibrant, healthy life. *Diet for Divine Connection* is not just information though. The teachings in this book embody the consciousness of Dr. Paul's deep knowing of having lived a life committed to understanding the interconnectedness she teaches. I'll be recommending this book to all of my clients!"

— Nancy Swisher, MA, MFA, author of *The Life That Woke Me Up Was My Own*, spiritual teacher, transformational coach, and certified Inner Bonding® facilitator

OTHER BOOKS BY MARGARET PAUL

Inner Bonding
Do I Have to Give Up Me to Be Loved By God?

WITH JORDAN PAUL, PHD
Do I Have to Give Up Me to Be Loved By You?
(over 1,000,000 copies sold)
Do I Have to Give Up Me to Be Loved By You? Workbook
Do I Have to Give Up Me to Be Loved By My Kids?

WITH ERIKA J. CHOPICH, PHD
Healing Your Aloneness
Healing Your Aloneness Workbook

DIET • FOR
divine
CONNECTION

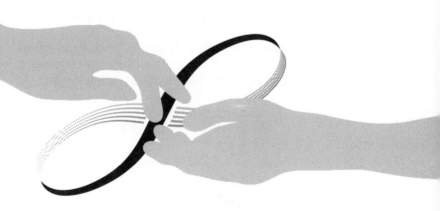

Beyond Junk Foods and Junk Thoughts
to At-Will Spiritual Connection

Margaret Paul, PhD

Best-Selling co-Author of
Do I Have to Give Up Me to Be Loved By You?
and *Healing Your Aloneness* and Author of *Inner Bonding*

© 2018 Margaret Paul
All rights reserved.

No part of this book may be used or reproduced in any manner without prior written permission from the publisher, except in the case of brief quotations embodied in critical reviews and articles.

The scanning, uploading, and distribution of this text via the Internet or any other means without the permission of the publisher is illegal and punishable by law. Please purchase only authorized electronic editions, and do not participate in or encourage electronic piracy of copyrighted materials. Your support of the author's rights is appreciated.

The information herein is for educational purposes only. The content of this book should not be used to give medical advice or to prescribe any form of treatment for physical, emotional, or medical problems without the advice of a physician, directly or indirectly. Should you use any recommendations in this book for yourself or others, the author, and the publisher assume no responsibility for your actions.

For information about special discounts for bulk purchases, please contact Light Technology Publishing Special Sales at 1-800-450-0985 or publishing@LightTechnology.net.

ISBN-13: 978-1-62233-060-7
ebook ISBN: 978-1-62233-795-8

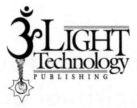

Light Technology Publishing, LLC
Phone: 1-800-450-0985
1-928-526-1345
Fax: 928-714-1132
PO Box 3540
Flagstaff, AZ 86003
LightTechnology.com

This book
is dedicated to
my Divine guidance, who
makes writing easy for me by
writing through me, who is always
here to guide me in my highest good
to help me manifest my passion and
purpose, and without whom I would
not know how to live and love. You
let me know in very many ways that
I am never alone, that you are
always here for me to lean on,
and that I can trust you
completely.

CONTENTS

Part 3 • Intention:
The Second Secret to Divine Connection
HEAL YOUR DIET OF JUNK THOUGHTS
AND UNLOVING ACTIONS AND LEARN TO LOVE YOURSELF

Part 4 • Action:
Use the Six Steps to Inner Bonding
ACHIEVE AT-WILL SPIRITUAL CONNECTION
TO HEAL YOURSELF PHYSICALLY, EMOTIONALLY, AND SPIRITUALLY

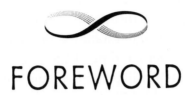

FOREWORD

It was thirty-six years ago that I was first introduced to Dr. Margaret Paul. At the time, I was looking for help with my personal life. The day I walked into her home office, I was greeted by a deeply compassionate, wise, and loving woman who I quickly came to see was also brilliant — and she has only become more so over the years.

From the moment we started our sessions together, it was clear that the friend who'd referred me to Dr. Paul had been entirely on the mark when she described her as an exceptional therapist. Dr. Paul was my first therapist, and the time spent with her proved extraordinarily helpful to me.

Fast-forward some years to my own work of helping others find deep and lasting happiness. Margaret's outstanding thirty-day Love Yourself Inner Bonding course has become an essential aspect of a program I teach called Your Miraculous Life. I've watched client after client use this process and heal old childhood wounds that had stopped them from showing up as the magnificent individuals they truly are. Margaret's Inner Bonding helps people establish an authentic connection with themselves, enabling them to move beyond a troubled past into a fulfilling and joyous present.

While I've found Dr. Paul's work to be immensely valuable in my own life and in the lives of my clients over the years, the aspect of transformation she brings into focus in *Diet for Divine Connection* fills a gap in our culture's understanding that's truly groundbreaking. I'm certain that her understanding of the link between our diet and our spiritual development will prove to be the missing piece for many who long to be happy and fulfilled in every dimension of their lives.

I'm particularly excited about this book because food and health have long been deep interests. I first stumbled across the connection between diet and a feeling of well-being in my mid-teens. Growing up, I had essentially existed on hot dogs and Ho Hos and the standard American diet, which appropriately carries the acronym SAD. In my teens, sad is what I was much of the time. Of course, I had absolutely no idea that my sadness and low-grade depression were in any way connected to my diet. But when I turned sixteen, I began the practice of meditation and simultaneously began eating more healthfully. As I did, the heavy blanket of sadness, inner emptiness, and disconnection started to lift.

But it wasn't until 1998 that the link between physical and spiritual well-being took center stage in my life. It was then that I began serious research into the literature on happiness. In addition to looking at the numerous studies that had been conducted in the field, I interviewed hundreds of people who were unconditionally happy. Gradually, I began incorporating the principles I was discovering into my personal life.

The change that made all the difference and really convinced me that I was on the right track came while I was in the throes of menopause. I was on a book tour for my newest book at the time, *Happy for No Reason*. It's not so great to be on tour for a book on happiness when you're as grumpy as I was! I knew I had to do something about the way I was feeling. I had been a sugar addict my entire life and was reluctant to give it up, but deep within I knew that I had to eliminate it from my diet.

In addition to going cold turkey on sugar, I dove into meditation in earnest — I had drifted away from the practice over the years — and started exercising again, another aspect of my life in which I had become lax. Within days, I witnessed the extraordinary correlation between how we treat our bodies and how we show up in life. I went from a moody, crazed, unhappy camper to a steady, calm, spiritually fulfilled person. Throughout the rest of the tour, I felt in integrity with promoting my book because the changes I had made rapidly shifted me back into my happy zone.

This is why when people come to me who are unhappy, one of the first things I tell them is to look at their diet. I have again and again witnessed the deep connection between what we eat and how we feel and live.

The message in this book is essential and timely. Sadly, one out of four women in North America is on antidepressants. This staggering epidemic of unhappiness is due in great part to these two things — our diet and our disconnection from our divine source. The way in which Margaret connects these two fields offers a quantum breakthrough in our understanding.

If ever I start to feel disconnected from my self-love, my divine connection, I turn to either Margaret's work or Margaret herself. She has proven to be a trusted guide over the decades. In this book, she will clearly show you how to use food and thought to strengthen your divine connection in a profound way.

— Marci Shimoff,
#1 NY Times best-selling author of
Happy for No Reason and *Love for No Reason*

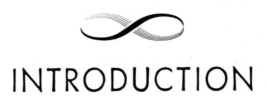

INTRODUCTION

Like so many people, I grew up in a dysfunctional family, and by the time I was five years old, I was a mess. I was an anxious nail biter with a persistent cough who had difficulty sleeping and experienced lots of nightmares. That's when my mother took me to a psychiatrist, whom I remember well.

After talking with me and with my mother, this tall, skinny man looked at me and told me to tell my mother not to yell at me. I clearly remember thinking, "I'm five years old. She isn't going to listen to me. Why don't *you* tell her?" And my next thought was, "I can do a better job than you." That's when I decided that I wanted to be a psychologist. I was the kind of empathic kid people came to with their problems, and I always loved helping.

I was not only a very anxious child but also very sickly. By my early twenties, I was tired of being sick. That's when I started to read everything I could about health and nutrition. After reading *Silent Spring* by Rachel Carson (Houghton Mifflin, 1962) and *The Poisons in Your Food* by William Longgood (Simon and Schuster, 1960), I threw all my food out and started to shop at the only health food store in Santa Monica, the Coop Market. As a result, my health greatly improved, and I've been eating only organic foods since. That was fifty-six years ago. I am now healthier than I've ever been and have extraordinary energy!

The Food and Thought Connection

My parents were atheists, so I grew up without religious or spiritual training. According to my father, anyone who believed in God was just using that as a crutch. I was a naturally spiritual child, but I completely suppressed it to fit into my family.

When I was in my early thirties, after my third child was born, I became interested in Divine connection. I tried everything — including following a guru, attempting various forms of meditation, and listening to tapes on opening up to channeling — but I couldn't seem to find the connection that I intuitively knew was available. Since my late teens, I had been in and out of therapy, trying every form of emotional healing available to me. It was also at this time that I earned my PhD in psychology.

I practiced for seventeen years as a traditional psychotherapist, and I was not at all happy with the results — not for my clients or me. That's when I started to pray for a process that would truly work to heal pain and bring joy.

In 1984, I met Dr. Erika Chopich, who helped me cocreate Inner Bonding. We each had half the process, so of course we had to meet! The six steps of the Inner Bonding process are as follows:

> **Step 1:** Be willing to feel pain and take responsibility for your feelings
> **Step 2:** Move into the intent to learn
> **Step 3:** Dialogue with your wounded and core selves
> **Step 4:** Dialogue with your higher guidance
> **Step 5:** Take loving action
> **Step 6:** Evaluate your action

As Dr. Chopich and I developed the six steps of the Inner Bonding process, which includes a spiritual connection, we realized that a vital aspect of spiritual connection is about intention — which you will learn about in this book. Once I was able to raise my frequency by consciously choosing my intention, I was instantly able to connect with my Divine source of love and wisdom.

I thought that everyone would be able to connect the way I did, but I was wrong. That's when I realized it was the combination of my food diet and my thought diet that raised my frequency high enough to easily connect. So I'm very excited to share with you how and why junk foods and "junk thoughts" prevent Divine connection and how a healthy food-and-thought diet will enable you to easily attain at-will Divine connection.

— Margaret Paul, PhD

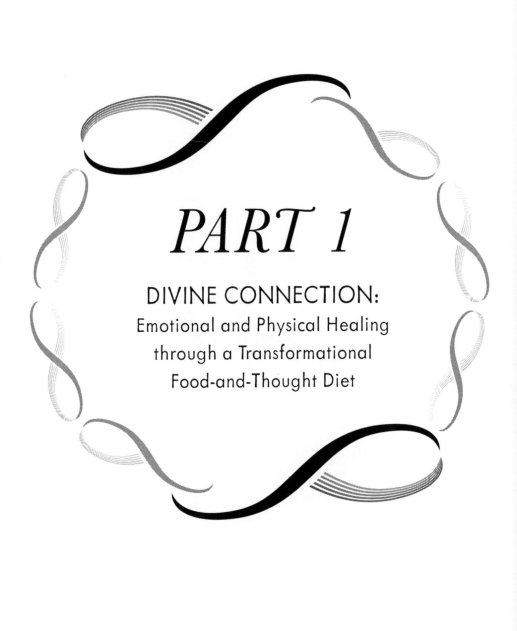

PART 1

DIVINE CONNECTION:
Emotional and Physical Healing through a Transformational Food-and-Thought Diet

CHAPTER 1

TAKE PERSONAL RESPONSIBILITY FOR YOUR HEALTH

The processed food industry, Big Pharma, and insurance companies are intricately linked to why we have both a spiritual crisis and a healthcare crisis in America. For example, my client Carrie was brought up by parents who knew nothing about nutrition. Both worked and had little time to cook, so they often relied on cheap meals from fast-food places such as McDonald's. The mother, frazzled and trying her best to take care of the family, often gave Carrie and her two brothers candy bars and cookies to get them off her back. Breakfast was sugary dry cereal with pasteurized milk.

As an adult, Carrie is addicted to packaged and processed food, especially those that contain high fructose corn syrup, which is in many foods and is partly responsible for the obesity problem in our country as well as many other serious illnesses that result from inflammation. The few fruits and vegetables she eats are canned or frozen and treated with pesticides and preservatives. The meat she eats from the factory farms is filled with antibiotics. Overweight and suffering from type 2 diabetes, Carrie was recently diagnosed with breast cancer.

Carrie wasn't taught that she is responsible for her health and well-being. Neither was she taught that she is mostly what she eats. She doesn't know that the food she is eating not only has little nutritional value but also is harming her. The large corporations that produce the food she eats don't want her to know that it's making her sick. They don't want her to know that the animal protein she consumes is so far from natural that it is harming her. They don't want her to know that the enriched, packaged foods are robbing her body of necessary nutrients.

The drug companies want Carrie to think that all she has to do is take a pill to make things better. They have no desire for her to know what's really happening when she takes their pills, and they certainly have no interest in her becoming responsible for her health and well-being. Sadly, many physicians, not to mention the insurance companies, also don't want patients to take responsibility for their health.

The bottom line of the health care crisis is greed. How can our government strongly encourage people to eat well and learn how to deal with their stress in responsible, nonaddictive ways and avoid harmful drugs when the corporations that put our leaders in power are the very ones who will lose money if people take responsibility for their health and well-being? Will these vast food, pharmaceutical, and insurance companies voluntarily give up their huge profits to advocate personal responsibility?

So Carrie enters the "health care" system, which charges a fortune to deal with her diabetes and cancer, both of which are degenerative diseases that can generally be prevented and even cured with foods that heal.[1, 2] When most think about their health, it's usually in terms of something having gone wrong. "Health care" has become a cipher for doctors, hospitals, pharmaceuticals, and the like, all of which are tailored to treat diseased and degenerative states. Consequently, as

---

1.   To learn more about how foods can heal, see FoodasMedicineInstitute.com.
2.   Charlotte Gerson, *The Gerson Therapy: The Proven Nutritional Program for Cancer and Other Illnesses* (New York City: Kensington Publishing, 2001).

more people suffer debilitating illnesses that require ongoing medication, expensive surgeries, and a growing demand for long-term care as a result of aging populations, the health care systems of country after country are experiencing unprecedented strain.

Based on repairing damage instead of avoiding it in the first place — despite the way we tip our hats to checkups, preventative care, and the like — the entire medical system is bowed under the weight of sickness caused by a food supply that, to a very large degree, is all but guaranteed to make us sick. Never has there been a greater need to think in terms not just of healing or even taking the usual preventative measures but also of enhancing health by means of a deep connection to that essential aspect of our humanity that's capable of offering us guidance on a person-by-person, moment-by-moment basis.

Even as our sophisticated technological approach to health care struggles under the burden of enormous costs, paradoxically never before have we been able to peer so deeply into the mechanisms by which high-quality foods optimize the effectiveness of the immune system through anti-inflammatory activity, elevating our experience of well-being. At the same time, the evidence that most of the food served up for our consumerist society is of inferior, health-damaging quality is readily available. We now know precisely how so many of the prepared foods found on grocery store shelves, particularly junk food, create imbalances in the human body, leading to many of the illnesses and degenerative diseases that threaten to break the bank.

Your Well-Being Is Your Responsibility

When you look at how the nation's health care system is set up, you see that it's geared toward the doctors, hospitals, and pharmaceutical companies that treat people only when they become ill, with minimal mention of prevention — let alone the idea that people should take responsibility for their own health and wellness. If it weren't such a lucrative industry, I wonder how much of the system would be around after people started adopting more economical preventative self-care. Yes, there are well-intended medical practitioners, and they are to be applauded. But as a whole, the system fosters personal irresponsibility and dependence on the so-called experts.

I believe that today people need to awaken to be responsible for their personal well-being and to connect with their capacity for Divine guidance so that they know how to take helpful action for themselves. With this in mind, I wish to conclude this chapter with a real-life example of how we escape responsibility — and a challenge to take charge of your health!

My client Sam works much harder in his retail business than either of his two partners and often feels overwhelmed by the amount he has to do. In this way, he's typical of many people in today's society who are used to a helter-skelter pace.

On weekends Sam doesn't relax and recuperate. Instead, he ends up doing work around the house even though he has two strong teens who could help out. When others offer to help, he turns them down — a surefire recipe for developing a martyr complex.

Most of us are decent people who are nice to know. Sam takes this a step further. Devoted to appearing to be a nice guy, he's constantly doing for others what they need to do for themselves.

Entirely in the shadow in this scenario is the fact that Sam is addicted to controlling how others perceive him. If someone doesn't acknowledge what a caring person he is, he feels irritated and taken advantage of. He will often obsessively ruminate about how unjust his wife and partners are.

Once Sam is upset, since he can't stand to feel this way, he has to drown his feelings in alcohol — even though he hates the hangovers that follow and knows that drinking too much is bad for his health. Others turn to junk food, binge eating, pharmaceuticals, or other methods of coping with their feelings.

When we fail to make a firm decision to take responsibility for our well-being, we become dependent on others to do it for us, which is what so much of the health care system is focused on. Once we hand over to others the responsibility of our worth, lovability, and safety, we inevitably do all we can to control them so that they supply us with what we think we need in order to feel worthy, happy, and safe. Hence, we have entire government organizations that seek to regulate and control our food supply, often making decisions that are far from our best interests.

From the Food and Drug Administration to the Center for Disease Control, others are intent on controlling what we put into our bodies in the form of food, pharmaceuticals, or vaccinations. It's time for everyone to face this fundamental truth: There isn't one person on the planet who actually wants the responsibility for your sense of worth and safety, just as you don't want that responsibility for other adults. People want to control you, yes. But that's the opposite of taking responsibility.

The present "health care" system is misnamed; it's more about profit and control than about well-being. If you didn't receive appropriate care as a child — which is the foundation of all authentic health care — it's too late for someone to do it for you; all you will get is control, the intent of which will be to benefit someone else. This is why you need to learn to responsibly care for yourself. Others can encourage you, but they can't do it for you. Only you are inside your body 24/7 with your feelings.

Your intent is what ultimately controls your actions. You won't be able to take responsibility for what you eat and drink unless you have addressed this aspect of your lives. Therefore, it's helpful to recognize the ways you make others responsible for your feelings — how you dump your feelings on to them. Ask yourself whether you have done any of the following:

- "I yell at, criticize, or blame, hoping the other person will understand how much I'm hurting and change what he or she is doing."
- "I calmly complain about something repeatedly, gently badgering the other person with the hope that he or she will say just the right thing to release the painful feelings in me. I believe that if this person agrees, changes, or acknowledges what he or she is doing, I will feel better. Even if the person does say the 'right' thing, I keep at it because it's never right enough."
- "I cry as a pathetic victim, hoping the other will feel badly enough to give me the compassion I'm not giving myself or that the person will stop doing what he or she is doing that's hurting me so that I don't have to take loving action for myself."
- "I talk on and on, hoping that if I talk enough and get enough attention from the other person, my pain will go away."
- "I shut down and withdraw from others, hoping they will feel badly enough to change and give me the understanding and compassion I'm not giving myself."

- "I have sex with my partner to release my stress and validate myself."

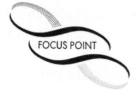

FOCUS POINT

Consider the effects any addictive behaviors you express have on your relationships. They are self-rejecting, and while they might work temporarily, they result in more disconnection.

What happens in your relationships when you engage in any of these addictive forms of behavior? While these self-rejecting tactics might work temporarily to distract you from your pain, they result in even more disconnection and loneliness between you and those important to you. While it might seem as if the pain subsides when you dump your feelings on others, all that really happens is that the feelings become more deeply entrenched until they are eventually stuck in your body, where they trigger physical and emotional problems.

It's pretty difficult to feed the body or the mind a Divine diet as long as we reject ourselves in such ways. This is why the process — Inner Bonding — that I use with my clients is so important. It goes to the heart of our diet issues, the heart of what it means to experience Divine connection.

CHAPTER 2

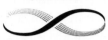

FOOD AND
DIVINE CONNECTION

The spirit being Ananda points out, "Always eat and think for the best and clearest energy and then the connection to Source and pathways to the Divine will open."[1] Many of us have heard that ancient gurus used to fast on mountaintops to access spiritual guidance. They knew that food and spirituality are connected and that cleansing the body would raise their vibrancy high enough to connect with their Divine source.

Some ancient cultures, including Native Americans, made ample use of food, especially herbs, in their rituals and ceremonies.[2] Much thought was given to the foods and herbs in death rituals and afterlife

1. Ananda through Tina Louise Spalding, *Making Love to God* (Flagstaff: Light Technology Publishing, 2013) p. 87.
2. See the following websites for more information on how Native Americans use plants and herbs in rituals and ceremonies:
    www.legendsofamerica.com/na-ceremonies/2/#Green%20Corn%20Festivals,
    https://en.wikipedia.org/wiki/Navajo_medicine,
    http://nativeamericannetroots.net/diary/951

rituals. The Navajo used herbs such as Utah juniper, broom snake-weed, and soapweed. Some tribes, believing that the energy of the food offered blessings, prepared food and decorated their houses with ears of corn to bless the dead. Tribes such as the Iroquois, Cherokee, and Seminole used corn in green corn ceremonies. These tribes would feast or fast in their spiritual ceremonies, and the corn was eaten only after the Great Spirit had been thanked for ripening the crops. Purifying the body was often a part of these ceremonies. It seems that people who lived close to nature intuitively understood how to increase their vibrancy.

Many Native American spiritual ceremonies also included herbs and plants as remedies to create a connection with spirits. Their spiritual rituals included tobacco, red cedar, sweetgrass, and sage. Many tribes combined spirituality, rituals, and herbal medicine as part of their healing practices. Such peoples didn't think of healing as curing disease but as making people whole, raising their vibrancy so that spirit — coursing through every cell, every molecule in their bodies — could heal them.

Purifying and cleansing also occurred in sweat lodges, where an ill person was often given sacred plants and herbal remedies while a healer worked to release low levels of vibrancy (understood as angry spirits) and invited the high vibrancy of healing spirits. Today we know that anger, anxiety, and depression lower our vibrancy and can cause illness, whereas higher levels of vibrancy, such as peace, joy, love, and compassion can, contribute to healing.

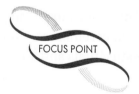

FOCUS POINT

Anger, anxiety, and depression lower our vibrancy and can cause illness, whereas peace, joy, love, and compassion can contribute to healing.

Vision quests were part of the practices of many Native American tribes, especially for adolescent boys moving into adulthood. People on vision quests often fasted as part of their preparation to connect with their spiritual guidance and find direction for their lives.

In most cultures, food is considered a sacred source of energy and nourishment — a source of life. Food and life are deeply entwined, as are food and vibrancy. It's sad that today food and eating are often experienced as stressful rather than as a sacred form of nourishing our bodies and sustaining health and wellness.

Despite the decline of mainstream religion in Western societies, more people than ever express an interest in exploring spirituality as a path to a more meaningful life. In tandem with this growing interest in life as a spiritual journey, large numbers are turning away from the traditional American diet and embracing what they regard as a more compassionate approach to food, one they deem healthier for the planet and for their bodies.

The principal forms of this shift away from meals built around meat, potatoes, bread, and iceberg lettuce with a wedge of tomato and slice or two of cucumber thrown in are vegetarian and vegan diets. Variations place an emphasis on consuming most foods in a raw state and avoiding grains, along with other permutations of what many deem a more spiritual lifestyle.

One Size Does Not Fit All

Despite this revolution in eating habits, I'm finding there's a striking lack in understanding how a one-size-fits-all approach to health care can be detrimental to our well-being and spiritual development. Most nutritional plans focus on foods that a particular food guru (and in some cases the government) tells us we ought to eat — often with an emphasis on what we shouldn't eat. This does little to help us heal the body so that body, mind, and soul can align. It's when our entire being is in alignment — every aspect of our humanity in balance — that we can develop the higher states of consciousness people are increasingly in search of.

Expanding our ability to make and sustain better food choices creates a context in which we are more able to change those habits that divorce us from the awareness that resides in our centers. In this way, high-quality nutrition supports our spiritual advancement.

In my practice of helping people individually, as couples, and in groups, I constantly come across clients whose diets are based on a chosen philosophy instead of on personal insight from Divine guidance. Again and again I see how this not only limits their attempt to function from a spiritual state with a high level of consciousness but also undermines their health and well-being — and thus their capacity for a spiritual connection.

A philosophy of eating and drinking is fundamentally different from being attuned to our unique personal requirements, the particularities of which become clear to us when we dive deeply enough into our spiritual connection with the Divine. When a philosophy rules us, whether adopted as a mindset or inspired emotionally, we simply cannot become aware of the deeper knowing that comes from Spirit. Nor are we in a place to recognize this knowing in others, whose different makeups and circumstances might require an approach to food that doesn't conform to our philosophies. When this occurs, the tendency to categorize, criticize, and condemn arises.

Vegans judge flesh eaters as cruel and view them as damaging their health, arguing that one should do nothing that causes the suffering of another creature. Vegetarians deem vegans too extreme. Those who consume a Paleo diet castigate vegans as squeamish and unhealthy. Anyone who doesn't see things "our" way is viewed as not spiritual.

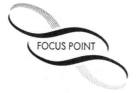

FOCUS POINT

When we are in tune with our guidance, we know what food is right for us in any given moment.

Labeling, and buying into a label, is fundamentally different from live, on-the-spot guidance from Divine connection. When we are in tune with our guidance, we know what's right for us in any given moment, no matter whose opinions it might violate.

To be healthy and enjoy robust well-being, high vibrancy, and ongoing access to our Divine guidance, we need to know specifically what to eat, what to drink, how to dispel stress, how to heal addiction, what forms of exercise and activity are right for us individually, and how to engage life in a way that's personally beneficial instead of run-of-the-mill.

One problem is that the ego is terrified of opening up and surrendering to the guidance that comes from our souls within and spirit around us, as the ego is addicted to the beliefs we were brought up with, the advice of peers and professionals, and the ways our culture (or the whole world) "does things." How dare we go against the conventional wisdom or what our peer groups endorse!

An important distinction exists between the intention to amass knowledge and the intention to experience the kind of internal knowing that comes as guidance. The intention to increase our knowledge can be purely ego, as it seeks to understand what to do and how to do it "right" so as to have control over getting what we want.

Few seem to inquire deep within concerning the optimization of their intake of food and beverages. Given the availability of mass communication and the ease of disseminating information in a manner unimaginable in any other era of human existence, it's helpful to consider different ideas about what we should or shouldn't eat. And there are countless conflicting ideas out there. In the end, it comes down to how what we choose to ingest affects our personal capacity for awareness, our health, and our behavior.

Food and the Environment

It ought to be common knowledge by now that not only our individual health and degree of consciousness are influenced by the quality of the foods we consume but also all aspects of the biosphere. Sadly, only a minority of humans seems aware that what we put into our bodies — and what we do to the environment to enable us to do this — has an impact on everyone.

Today the hormones from contraceptive pills, antibiotics fed to animals, artificial fertilizers and pesticides applied to crops, and countless chemicals used in the manufacturing process of foods and other goods are turning up in our lakes, rivers, and oceans. Just how low a level of consciousness we operate at as a species is especially evident in the fact that our government must warn us that eating certain amounts of fish can expose us to toxic levels of mercury. But what are they doing to stop the mercury contamination? Has anyone figured out how to remove mercury from the vast oceans that feed us? Has anyone considered how to remove the glyphosates (broadspectrum herbicides used to rid our farms of weeds) from the food chain?

How much more unaware can we be when it comes to understanding how to foster vibrant health and a general feeling of well-being? How powerful are these assets in terms of enjoying the kind of spiritual connection that transforms everyday life from a mundane, mediocre experience to an adventure that's simply magnificent?

Food of the Gods

Haven't we all at some time remarked while devouring a scrumptious dessert, chocolate, or ice cream, "Mmm, this is simply divine"? For thousands of years, humans of every culture have thought of certain foods earth produces for our enjoyment as food of the gods. The ancient Greek myths, for instance, speak of ambrosia as a food of the Greek gods: It has the ability to bestow longevity and even immortality on those who consume it.

The pantheon of ancient gods was long ago superseded by more-informed views, so few of us in the modern world think in terms of gods consuming sacred foods.

Yet even in the era of monotheism, the Jewish tradition features a banquet in which the Hebrew God Yahweh feasts with his people, and the Christian faith has as its focal point a symbolic meal referred to originally as a love feast. It seems we can't escape the link between food and the Divine.

With all the information about food that's available today, how can you know what's best for your health and vibrancy? When so much of the advice is contradictory, whose guidance can you rely on? How can you be sure someone isn't feeding you biased information that's going to end up harming you?

For a while there has been a movement away from gluten among some who seek to be in tiptop health. Gluten is found in grains such as wheat, barley, and rye. Many people have shifted instead to different forms of carbohydrates, including quinoa, millet, buckwheat, oats, and rice, in particular. Now we're being told that much of the rice we consume contains damaging quantities of arsenic. It's a case of damned if you do and damned if you don't.

Then there's the matter of eggs, which for the past three decades have been castigated for dumping bad cholesterol into our bloodstreams. Only it turns out that cholesterol isn't exactly the cause of heart attacks, and eggs are actually healthy for most people, as long as they are from free-range chickens given organic feed.[3] We are now being informed that eggs don't raise a person's cholesterol and can in fact be a balanced and healthy choice — unless of course you are allergic to them or follow a vegan diet.

Recent research also shows that cholesterol has nothing to do with heart disease. On the contrary, we're now told that we need the good fats that foods such as eggs provide and that eliminating them is one of the causes of the rise in Alzheimer's.[4] Meanwhile, other leaders in the health field tell us that even organic, pastured eggs are not healthy for us for a variety reasons.[5]

Should you eat potatoes? Nah, surely they're just carbohydrates and cause you to put on weight. Really? It turns out that there's such a thing as resistant starch, and if potatoes are prepared in the appropriate way, they act on the body quite differently.[6]

The number of foods and beverages we could list that have at one time been considered beneficial and no longer are or have been regarded as harmful and are now known to be good for us is extensive. Since the recommendations are changing as research is conducted and our understanding deepens, how can we know what's part of a healthy diet and what isn't, especially as advertising blasts are presented to us as the truth? I'm providing the following story as an example of just one approach to what we should or shouldn't eat.

Seated around a table at a resort dedicated to health and spirituality, a group of guests listened intently as a yogi explained why, when

3. More information can be found about this subject at https://www.mind-bodygreen.com/articles/are-eggs-healthy.

4. Dr. David Perlmutter, *Brain Maker* (Boston: Little, Brown and Company, 2015). pp. 13, 72, 221.

5. Dr. Amy Myers, *The Autoimmune Solution* (San Francisco: HarperOne, 2017) pp. 77, 114, and 183, and Anthony William, *Medical Medium* (Carlsbad: Hay House, 2015) pp. 132. 280–281.

6. Learn about resistant starch at http://drhyman.com/blog/2016/03/24/the-starch-that-makes-you-lean-and-healthy/.

ordering dinner, he had requested that the chef use no garlic, onions, ginger, or leeks in the preparation of the dish he had selected.

The young yogi said, "Each of the many different kinds of foods the earth provides has a unique frequency or vibrational pattern. Some foods have a high frequency, others a more moderate frequency, and some an especially low frequency. Long ago, the yogic tradition discovered that the particular vibration of a food has a profound impact on our health and well-being, as well as on the depth of the connection we experience to the Divine."

A young woman from Australia interrupted and inquired of the yogi, "Presumably you deem garlic, onions, ginger, and leeks to be of a very low vibration?"

"Indeed," said the yogi, "which is why I prefer not to eat them. Their vibration is among the lowest of all foods."

"What effect do they have on you when you consume them?" a man from India, who looked to be in his seventies, asked.

"They stimulate desire," said the yogi.

Noticing that the young yogi was extremely handsome, the Australian pressed, "So what's wrong with desire?"

"You understand that I'm speaking not of the desire one might have for oneness with the Divine or what many in the West refer to as God. I'm speaking of the kind of desire that's connected with the baser urges of the species."

"You mean sex," the young woman quipped.

"Ah," said the older man, "given that you are a yogi and committed to a celibate life, that makes sense. So no garlic, onion, ginger — and presumably other spices — for you! But for those of us who have learned that Divine sex can be a path to Divine connection, garlic, onion, leeks, and ginger might be helpful rather than hurtful!"

An older woman with an American accent joined the discussion, inquiring, "What exactly do you mean by 'vibration'?"

"Everything in the universe vibrates," the yogi explained enthusiastically. "Not just living things but also the rocks, sand, and dirt. We can measure this vibration in hertz. The vibration of one kind of food is different from that of another. Like garlic and onions, animal flesh is of a low vibration, as is dairy, whereas most fruit and vegetables are much higher."

"I know what hertz are, of course," the American responded. "We're speaking of how you measure frequency such as in the case of sound waves, light waves, or electromagnetic radiation. But tell me, have you actually measured these food frequencies you speak of? And how would you go about doing so?"

"I haven't measured the frequency of any foods personally," the yogi admitted, "although I've heard you can use a pendulum. In my case, I don't concern myself with measurements because the yogic tradition has known for thousands of years which foods vibrate at higher frequencies and are beneficial versus which are less beneficial or even injurious to our health and well-being."

A man who had remained silent until this point spoke with an accent that was distinctly French. "Well, I'm a biologist by profession," he launched in, "and I can tell you for a certainty that the idea of measuring a food's vibration, or frequency, as you call it, has no basis in science. But I'm not entirely unfamiliar with the concept, given that my sister is a follower of a New Age guru and lives in a commune where they raise all their own food organically. They don't consume meat, poultry, fish, or any dairy, having apparently ascertained that such foods are of a 'low vibration,' as you say. They actually take everything a step beyond a vegetarian diet, even beyond a vegan diet, believing that to attain a high spiritual state as well as optimum physical health, everything must be ingested in its raw form. But I'm very skeptical because many in her community are not at all healthy! I've heard that some even believe they will ultimately be able to transcend all need for eating or drinking of any kind, existing simply on their breath!"

"Ah," chimed in the Australian, "so they are a group of would-be airheads!"

"Gosh," chuckled the Indian man in his seventies. "Where's the pleasure in life if you can't enjoy a good meal with friends? Surely it's possible to eat and drink for enjoyment and still be healthy?"

"To be spiritual too," insisted the American. "I'm a firm believer that, far from being the antithesis of what it means to live a spiritual life, healthy food enjoyed in an atmosphere of conviviality has an uplifting, beneficial effect on not only the body but also the mind and emotions. I'm equally convinced that the judging, nitpicking, and shaming that goes on where food is concerned in a lot of these sup-posedly spiritual movements is anything but health giving."

The French biologist leaned back in his chair, appearing pen-sive as he took a sip of mango juice. "Even though I don't necessarily support the 'frequency of foods' concept, there is a truth to the idea that some foods increase the vibrancy of our health, whereas others degrade our physical well-being — along with dulling us mentally, emotionally, and spiritually."

Health and Spiritual Well-being: Not a New Concept

That the state of our physical health affects our ability to experi-ence Divine connection isn't a modern idea, let alone the sole prov-ince of New Age groups. There is an increasing number of scientists who are connecting the fields of health and spiritual well-being.[7] You realize just how ancient this take on health and spirituality is if you search back in history a few thousand years.

There's an abundance of evidence that the major traditions from the Chinese, Indian, and ancient Greek civilizations conceived of health not only in terms of our physical states but also our emo-tional and spiritual states. They knew that the state of our health affects our ability to think clearly, our capacity for feeling deeply, our aptness to connect with one another, and the degree to which we perceive our connection to the universe. If we cut through all the elaborate conceptualizing with respect to the body and soul (which makes the topic of health and spirituality appear complex), we see that at the core of each tradition is an awareness that, to be in excellent health, substances flowing or being transported within the body must do so unimpeded and in just the right balance with the whole organism in harmony. As those who study medical sci-ence are increasingly coming to understand, the idea is that disease occurs when this flow is disrupted, which creates an imbalance in the body and results in a state of disharmony that renders us ripe for the development of a diseased organism as well as for contract-ing infection from our surroundings.

---

7. For some examples of this, see http://www.mdpi.com/2077-1444/2/1/17 and https://www.ncbi.nlm.nih.gov/pmc/articles/PMC1305900/.

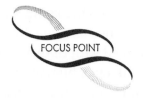

FOCUS POINT

The ancient Chinese, Indians, and Greeks knew that the state of our health affects our ability to think clearly, our capacity for feeling deeply, our aptness to connect with one another, and the degree to which we perceive our connection to the universe.

A remarkable aspect of the ancient Chinese, Indian, and Mediterranean traditions is that despite their superficial differences, they were consistent in recognizing that a major aspect in creating good health results from a balance of nutritional substances. They also regard each person as an integrated whole, not as a collection of separate parts, each like a machine. This is the opposite of the predominant mindset of Western medicine, which until recently subscribed to the view that the human organism is a conglomeration of separate mechanisms to be tinkered with in the way we tinker with our automobiles when some part goes haywire. Many of you might have had the frustrating experience of going to a doctor only to be sent to one specialist after another with none of them treating you as an integrated whole.

A further commonality among the Chinese, Indian, and ancient Greek traditions is each promotes the notion that an organism has the ability to heal itself through high-quality foods. This is a viewpoint that's only lately beginning to receive attention in scientific research — with Western medicine's gold standard of double-blind studies that it justly deserves. This reminds me of a famous quote by Hippocrates: "Let food be thy medicine and medicine be thy food."

The three principal ancient traditions were not alone in understanding that our physicality cannot be separated from the spiritual state. From time immemorial, ancient people the world over have shown some level of awareness of the intimate bond between physical well-being and what, in their understanding, they deemed to be the realm of the gods. Despite their lack of sophistication, they intuited at least the essence of what today our test tubes and microscopes are revealing.

Today, thanks to the advent of innovative technology, a rift that has existed for the past several centuries is slowly closing. Ever since the scientific revolution that began with such towering geniuses as Copernicus, Kepler, Descartes, and Newton, science and spirituality have tended to be at odds. This rift was exacerbated with the arrival of Darwin. A populace that was accustomed to thinking of human beings as discrete parts — body and soul, or body, mind, and spirit — had a tough time embracing these familiar terms as descriptions of a single entity rather than imagining one as housed inside the other.

Now, after centuries of alienation from one another, we are witnessing the beginnings of a merging of science and spirituality in a transformative way that's assisting us in understanding the importance of an integrated approach to health and well-being in which spirituality functions as a linchpin.

CHAPTER 3

DIVINE GUIDANCE IS AVAILABLE TO YOU

What if you knew that you are never alone? How would life be different for you if you had an ongoing, two-way communication with a divine source of love, compassion, wisdom, and guidance? This is available for you if you know how to access it, and this book offers two profound secrets to attaining this connection.

Everyone is a part of the field of intelligence known as the Divine. There are numerous names that people use for the Divine, such as God, Goddess, Spirit, Higher Power, Great Spirit, the All, or the Universe. I use these terms interchangeably to refer to the underlying intelligence, love, and inspiration found throughout creation. Manifested as intuition or inner knowing, Divine connection serves as a means of personal guidance. You can learn to tap into this guidance, which enables you to know what is in your highest good at any given moment.

In *The Biology of Belief* (Hay House, 2008), Bruce H. Lipton explains how all the cells in the body are informed by an intelligence that undergirds the entire creation, exerting its influence universally, which is also seen in the structure of galaxies and the makeup of atoms. Biologists have witnessed some powerful demonstrations of this intelligence at work. In his excellent book, *One Mind* (Hay House, 2014), Dr. Larry Dossey sites studies that demonstrate the power of universal intelligence. For example, in studies with twins who were separated at birth and had no knowledge of each other, they frequently, unconsciously name their children the same names as their twins, dress similar to their twins, and even marry partners with the same names!

The exciting aspect of this is that other sources have begun to link the vibrancy of the foods we consume, the thoughts we think, and our health in general with our ability to connect with Divine guidance.[1] Our level of vibrancy, or frequency, is essential for having a finely attuned level of awareness, a knowing that we can tap into what's within and all around us. In other words, what we experience as our inner compass is simultaneously the intelligence evident in every aspect of the universe.

When I discovered the amazing source of spiritual guidance flowing from deep within and all around me, I began to understand that instead of having to rely solely on the opinions of experts — which entailed sorting through a plethora of contradictory opinions and in the end siding with one viewpoint or the other (essentially guessing which piece of research is correct) — I could discover the answers I needed by tapping into both my inner and outer spiritual sources of knowing.

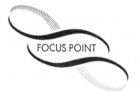

FOCUS POINT

Instead of relying completely on the advice of experts, tap into your inner and outer sources of knowing to discover the answers you need.

I don't mean to imply that research isn't valuable. I have researched much of what I understand about health and wellness, going into the various studies and expert opinions and interpretations of the data in considerable depth. But what I've come to see is that if I'm to be physically and emotionally healthy and enjoy a high degree of well-being,

---

1.   Ananda through Tina Louise Spalding in *Spirit of the Western Way* (Flagstaff: Light Technology Publishing, 2016) p. 37.

I need to know whether something that seems beneficial for most people is actually beneficial for me.

Is it right for my unique makeup, mindset, and situation? This is what the guidance that communicates through our deepest being, and through what some of us speak of as our highest selves, could show me. Whichever terminology you prefer, it's this field of love and intelligence, experienced personally as well as universally, that I have in mind when I use the term "Divine."

A Greater Understanding of the Term "God"

When I use the term "Divine connection," I'm not referring to traditional ideas about God or the practices of religion. I'm referring specifically to our ability to connect with the love and intelligence that manifests in everything. Today, more people are aware that using the term "God" doesn't require imagining a being seated on a kingly throne above the sky. Most of us think more in terms of a Divine reality that, as the psalmist puts it, "fills heaven and earth," or as St. Paul expressed, "In him [God] we live, and move, and have our being" [Acts 17:28, KJV]. I am also speaking of the love that is God, as expressed in 1 John 4:16 [NASB], "God is love, and he who abides in love abides in God, and God in him." It is my experience and the experience of the many thousands of people I've counseled that love is the foundation of universal intelligence.

In cultures across the planet, people are becoming aware of a higher order, a depth of consciousness, or a mysterious presence that pervades creation. This higher order, which I refer to as the Divine, encompasses everything. No aspect of the material world or the universe is separate from the Divine, as many of us today understand it.

When I refer to Divine connection, what I have in mind is a vital, fully alive, two-way connection with our source of love and wisdom. Call this God, or use whatever term works for you. Just be aware that while the ego — the false, damaged idea of ourselves we carry around in our heads — may believe in God, it does not know God and cannot experience Divine connection. The people we might imagine ourselves to be from our wounded egos cannot have a direct spiritual experience because we don't know who we are; we don't know our true selves. With no awareness of our true selves, we are closed to Divine connection.

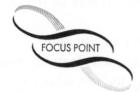

FOCUS POINT
Divine connection is a vital two-way exchange with our Source of love and wisdom.

To me, to be spiritual and divinely connected is to approach the whole of life from the background consciousness of the love and wisdom that is the Divine. We can draw on it for guidance in our personal lives while recognizing that we are all part of a matrix in which we are interconnected and to which the whole universe owes its existence.

Vibrancy Is Essential to Divine Connection

Nikola Tesla said, "If you want to find the secrets of the universe, think in terms of energy, frequency and vibration." Divine connection occurs when our vibrancy or frequency is high enough to make us energetically available to the higher vibration of Divine guidance. All matter is made up of energy. Energy vibrates, and the higher the vibration of the energy, the higher the frequency. All atoms, protons, and neutrons vibrate at particular frequencies. Everything in the universe has a vibrational frequency.

To put it more scientifically, "All matter vibrates at the molecular level, and every object possesses what is called a natural frequency, which depends on its size, shape, and composition.... Frequency in oscillation is the number of cycles per second, and in wave motion, it is the number of waves that pass through a given point per second. These cycles per second are called Hertz (Hz).... If something has a frequency of 100 Hz, this means that 100 waves are passing through a given point during the interval of one second, or that an oscillator is completing 100 cycles in a second. Higher frequencies are expressed in terms of kilohertz (kHz; 10^3 or 1,000 cycles per second); megahertz (MHz; 10^6 or 1 million cycles per second); and gigahertz (GHz; 10^9 or 1 billion cycles per second)."[2]

---

2. These excerpts are taken from ScienceClarified.com at http://www.science clarified.com/everyday/Real-Life-Physics-Vol-2/Frequency-How-it-works. html#ixzz4Oaik6wFS.

Simply put, frequency is how often an event repeats per second. The more oscillations that occur in a shorter period, the higher the vibration or frequency. An example for understanding frequency is a radio or a TV station. Each radio and TV station has a different frequency, which is what enables you to tune in to what you want to watch or listen to. When you want to tune in to a TV station, you turn to a particular channel, which has a particular frequency. Just because you can't see the radio or TV waves doesn't mean they aren't there. You accept their presence because the music or news you want to listen to comes through the radio and the show you want to see comes through the TV.

Just as you tune to a particular radio station or TV channel to connect with what you want to hear or see, you can learn to tune to a particular inner frequency — inner vibrancy — to connect with your personal source of Divine guidance, and this book teaches you how to do this. Just as you don't have to believe that the radio and TV waves are there because you experience the result of tuning in to your station, you don't have to believe that your Divine guidance is here for you. You will know this is true when you experience it.

Since no one has yet found a way to accurately measure human frequency (including the thoughts we think) or the frequency of the foods we eat, I mostly use the term "vibrancy" in place of "frequency" throughout this book. For example, eating at McDonald's is like putting a bell jar over your body. The low vibrancy of these processed foods (i.e., their low nutrient density) affects your level of vibrancy. Losing vibrancy makes it much harder to connect with Divine guidance.

Vibrancy is a central theme of this book. Having a low level of vibrancy is like having the electricity go out at night with no candles available. You're in the dark with no way of accessing the light. In this book, you will learn much about keeping your vibrancy high enough to connect with Divine guidance.

How It Feels to Connect with Divine Guidance

Have you ever experienced a moment when suddenly something became very clear to you? A moment when your heart felt warm and you felt full and peaceful inside, in sync and in tune with the world around you? A moment when you had a sense of oneness and connection with everything? Sometimes we call this moment grace, as suggested in the lyrics of the song "Amazing Grace": "I once was lost, but now am found / Was blind, but now I see." It's the difference between trying to see through a dirty or fogged up window and a very clean and clear window. We not only see things clearly but also feel a deep sense of joy and well-being, and we feel full of endless possibilities.

This is what it feels like when we are connected with Divine guidance. We feel an incredible sense of clarity about what is right and true for us, and we also feel a kind of inner peace that only comes when we are connected with Divine guidance. The poet William Wordsworth grasped what Divine connection feels like when, in "Tintern Abbey," he penned these lines:

And I have felt
A presence that disturbs me with the joy
Of elevated thoughts; a sense sublime
Of something far more deeply interfused,
Whose dwelling is the light of setting suns,
And the round ocean and the living air,
And the blue sky, and in the mind of man,
A motion and a spirit, that impels
All thinking things, all objects of all thought,
And rolls through all things.

In his words, we have a clear statement of what it means to be truly sentient, conscious, aware people whose existence is grounded in the Divine — which is how, from continent to continent, increasing numbers of us understand what it is to be spiritual. Before I discovered the two profound secrets to Divine connection that I will share with you, this experience of the grace of Divine connection used to happen to me occasionally. Now I have this experience most of the time, and you will too as you learn how to access your Divine guidance at will.

When I first started to access my Divine guidance, I was never sure whether the thoughts or images that popped into my mind were coming *from* my mind or *through* my mind. With practice, I learned to discern the difference in vibrancy between these two experiences.

I also learned that Divine guidance reveals itself in two ways. One is through our feelings, which always let us know whether we are coming from love and truth. The other is through the thoughts and images that pop into our minds. I know I'm on the right track when my thoughts and feelings line up. You will be learning much more about this in part 3.

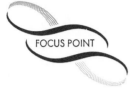

Divine guidance reveals itself through two areas: Our feelings, which always indicate whether we are coming from love and truth, and the thoughts and images that pop into our minds. When thoughts and feelings align, you're on the right track.

CHAPTER 4

HOW DIVINE CONNECTION WILL CHANGE YOUR LIFE

When I learned how to connect with Divine guidance and experience at-will, two-way communication, my life changed dramatically. I was no longer dependent on others and experts regarding what was right or wrong for me. I no longer had to run to therapists when life threw me a curve ball. I no longer stressed endlessly over important decisions. I no longer depended on others' approval. And true peace and joy no longer eluded me.

My powerful connection with Divine guidance didn't happen overnight. Like anything worth learning, it took practice, and I finally knew what to practice!

Decisions are now easy for me to make. I simply tune in to my Divine guidance, and very quickly I know what to do. Of course, it took time for me to trust my guidance — I had to test it over and over — but eventually I knew that I was never alone and that I was always being guided toward my highest good.

Another huge change was that I no longer needed to try to get love, compassion, or approval from others. Connecting with Divine guidance fills me with love to share with others, and all my relationships have improved as a result. My health has improved dramatically now that I know how to eat for my particular body to maintain a high vibrancy, and I know how to treat myself in loving ways — which goes very far in managing the stress in my life.

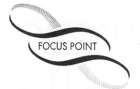

FOCUS POINT

When you are connected with the love and compassion of your Divine guidance, you will no longer need to try to get love, compassion, or approval from others.

Many people know that stress is implicated in the development of many illnesses, so learning how to manage stress in such nerve-racking times is vital to health, well-being, and vibrancy. Connecting with Divine guidance is essential for managing stress, and managing stress is vital in maintaining high vibrancy and Divine connection.

Creating heath, well-being, and vibrancy is less about gathering information than it is about tapping into our source of knowing. People can become addicted to gathering information, imagining it will give them more peace and more power. In contrast, opening ourselves to spiritual guidance means we know what's right for us at any given moment because we are being directed on a moment-by-moment basis. Our inner, higher self is an infallible guidance system, letting us know what's beneficial, harmful, right, or wrong for us. The following exchange with a client named April illustrates this:

"I want to share with you one of the ways in which my life has changed since I've been connecting with my inner guidance," April told me. "This might not sound momentous to you, but it's huge for me."

April explained how she always had difficulty making decisions, often making the wrong ones. "Before I started to work with you, when I was redecorating our living room, it took me forever to decide on a couch," she confided. "When I finally did and it arrived, I hated it."

"So what did you do?" I inquired.

"I suffered with it all year, but I finally decided to get a new one. Only this time, instead of trying to figure it out in my head, I tuned in to my heart and higher self."

"And?"

"It was an amazing experience to feel what I love. It's almost as if the right couch called to me. It might sound strange, but I could feel into the different couches, which is how I knew which was right for me."

"Did your couch arrive yet?" I asked, interested to know the outcome of this venture into the heart.

"It came two days ago," April enthused, "and I love it! I can't believe how easy the decision was this time. I'm so grateful to have discovered how to make decisions that are right for me."

Focused in her heart, with her body fully alive and attuned to the moment, April could perceive what she truly wanted in a couch. But it wasn't just her preferences for the type of couch that changed. Her feeling that she was one with her new couch spilled over into an awareness of the subtle information that's being broadcast everywhere all the time and can transform every aspect of our lives.

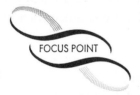

FOCUS POINT

When you are connected to your higher self, you know what's right at any time because you are directed moment by moment. Your inner self and higher self is infallible.

Authentic Guidance versus Ego Guidance

Without consciousness, it can be very easy to fool ourselves that we are being guided when what's leading us is really our wounded egos. When I think of being led by a wounded ego, I think of Glenn, a man who told his wife Cheryl that God was guiding him when he decided to have an affair as part of his spiritual journey. So many times have I heard that from people! In this case, he and his lover had gone a step further and were using drugs to connect with God. Neither of them was taking responsibility for their feelings at all (which you will learn to do in part 3). In fact, both had long histories of avoiding responsibility for both their pain and their joy, and the drugs were a way to continue to escape.

After opening up to her own pain about this situation and doing much inner work regarding her part in her relationship with Glenn, Cheryl decided to leave the marriage. She was deeply saddened to watch the man she loved avoid facing himself, but she realized that this had been his practice throughout their marriage.

Regardless of what you believe your inner guidance is telling you, if the result isn't peace and joy accompanied by loving action, it isn't coming from your Divine guidance but rather from your wounded ego. Authentic guidance always results in inner peace and joy as well as loving action for us and others, which is how we know we're on the right track. Our inner state is a sure barometer of what's really driving us. When you learn to stay tuned to your deep feeling states, you will know when you are truly guided and when your wounded ego is in charge.

Being able to make the best decisions for us is just one of the many results of living connected with Divine guidance. When we approach life from a highly present, vibrant, and aware state, we become far more attuned to everyone and everything. Instead of encountering people, things, and events on a surface level, we begin picking up their vibes. We tune in to the waves of energy that are all around us and moving through us. Things we just didn't notice before start popping out at us.

Ten Signs of Low Vibrancy

- You feel anxious, depressed, guilty, shamed, or miserable.
- You feel numb, heavy, or dead inside, as if you're just going through the motions in life.
- You feel alone and empty.
- Your focus is in your head rather than present in your body.
- You act out addictively with food, drugs, alcohol, sex/porn, shopping, spending, gambling, TV, internet, and so on.
- You are angry and critical, and you try to get someone else to make you feel safe, worthy, and lovable.
- You give yourself up, sacrificing yourself to get another's love and attention.
- You judge yourself or others.
- You lack a sense of purpose, and you don't know why you are on the planet.
- You can't connect with Divine guidance.

Ten Signs of High Vibrancy

- You feel peaceful and full inside.

- You revel in life, feeling light, happy, joyful, creative, optimistic, and enthusiastic.
- You feel genuine gratitude for your life and for big and small daily blessings.
- You are able to tap into Divine guidance regularly, and you feel connected to something bigger than you.
- You notice synchronicity.
- You feel a sense of passion and purpose.
- You feel compassionate and forgiving toward yourself and others, including others who have hurt you.
- You are present in your body, even with the painful feelings of life, such as loneliness, grief, helplessness concerning others, and heartbreak. You are able to lovingly embrace the painful feelings of life with compassion rather than avoid them with addictions.
- You never feel alone in the universe, and you know you are always being guided toward your highest good.
- You are easily able to manifest your dreams.

The Sound of Sheer Silence

When we are clear because we are following the kind of thought-and-food diet that facilitates awareness and vibrancy, we experience being guided. We intuit when someone is safe, dangerous, authentic, or deceptive. We can make decisions easily because we feel what's right for us. We know things without knowing how we know them.

My experience is that I am able to receive the exact input I need at any given moment, often only a moment before it's needed. That way, I'm not overwhelmed with information, and only what I require at the time comes to me. As long as I'm open to learning and in a physically vibrant state, I receive exactly what I need.

In his book *One Mind*, Dr. Larry Dossey tells a story about a woman who dreamed she had breast cancer. Nothing showed up on her mammogram or in an examination, but she took loving action for herself and insisted on a biopsy, which turned out to be cancerous.

"The pathologist called the original doctor with the report. 'This is the most microscopic breast cancer I've seen,' he said. 'You could not have felt it. There would have been no signs or symptoms. How did you find it?'

"'I didn't,' he replied. 'She did. In a dream.'"[1]

This doesn't mean that all our dreams portend something that significant. However, an individual whose intuition is alive and well knows how to separate the wheat from the chaff. One key to separating the ego from intuition is to be aware that loud voices are generally the ego, whereas Divine guidance is generally quite subtle. This requires us to be truly present so that we are attuned to what our guidance is trying to show us.

Hebrew scriptures [in the book of Deuteronomy] contain a story that illustrates the difference between the external loudness and showiness of the ego and the quiet inner knowing of our authentic selves receiving Divine guidance. At a time when the prophet Elijah was experiencing a great deal of opposition and felt discouraged, he asked to see God. He was told to journey to Mount Horeb and to stand on the mountainside whereupon God would pass by.

The first thing to occur was a mighty wind that was so powerful it dislodged huge rocks that tumbled down the mountain and broke into pieces. But God wasn't in the wind. Following the wind, there was an earthquake, and still God didn't make an appearance. Then a fire-storm ensued, no doubt caused by an awesome display of lightning. Was God in the fire? Nope.

It was what happened next that's so insightful and relevant to our everyday lives. Absent any external signs, God's presence was made known in what the translators tend to describe as "a still, small voice." However, this is an inadequate representation of the intent of the Hebrew. The translation provided by the New Revised Standard Version [1 Kings 19:12] makes it intelligible: "a sound of sheer silence." It was in this complete stillness, this utter silence, this absolute peace, that the Divine was made known. When we are able to attain this inner stillness, the Divine is made known to us.

What if Elijah's vibrancy had been low due to stuffing himself with junk food and indulging in junk thoughts? Would he have been able to pierce through the low physical vibrancy or the junk thoughts or the resulting painful emotions and junk actions that

---

1.   Larry Dossey, MD, *One Mind* (Carlsbad: Hay House, 2014) p. 22.

prevent most of us from tapping into this Divine inner knowing?

When the body is clogged with foods and thoughts that don't promote serenity and clarity, the waves of information that are available whenever we need them pass right by us. The beautiful thing about this is that many of our young people are learning to tune in to their intuition early in life so that they don't have to go through unlearning a lot of bad habits and having to cleanse their bodies of the effects of a lousy food-and-thought diet. More parents are helping their children adopt the kind of foods and thoughts that facilitate Divine connection. One mother told me the following story:

> My son came to me the other day and said, "Mom, you know, since I've been on this diet, I've noticed more little things working out. Like the other day, I had left a reusable shopping bag in my locker at school, and when I went to leave for the day, I realized, 'How perfect. I needed this now to pack up and take home these other items.'" I reminded him it was not just that more things are working out, but it was also that he is mentally and emotionally clearer now and able to notice these coincidences, and this to me is the nature of being in touch with our intuition.
>
> I'm blessed that my daughter feeds my grandsons a diet fit for the Divine nature that is their essence because the alertness it fosters shows up in their heightened intuition. To illustrate, my grandson Everest was filling balloons with helium for his eighth birthday party, and he gave one to his friend Henry. As Henry walked outside with the balloon, Everest went to his mother (my daughter Sheryl), and said, "I don't want Henry to let go of the balloon. I don't want it to be lost."
>
> "I know you don't, sweetie," Sheryl responded, "and I'm quite sure Henry doesn't either." Trusting his intuition, Everest walked over to Henry and stood right next to him. Moments later, Henry accidentally let go of the balloon. Uh-oh! But I watched in amazement as Everest intuitively reached up and caught it! Henry looked at him with absolute delight as Everest handed the balloon back to him. Not wanting to risk losing it again, Henry took it inside.

"Wow, Everest," I remarked, "that was amazing!"

"Grandma, I think the force was with me," Everest responded. He was of course referring to *Star Wars*, which enthralled him at the time, as it did his little brother, through the comics their father reads to them.

"I'm so glad you trusted the force," I congratulated him, smiling as he grinned from ear to ear. "But how did you know Henry was going to let go of the balloon at exactly that second?"

"I can't explain it," he said. "I just knew."

I just knew — that's intuition. It's the insight that arises in situation after situation once we are attuned to "the sound of sheer silence" in which the Divine is made known.

Do you see how practical our guidance wishes to be in terms of our everyday lives? Even in the littlest things, Divine connection makes all the difference. It's what can inform us more accurately than anyone or anything of what's appropriate for us in terms of our diet, lifestyle, and everyday life decisions, as well as our safety and well-being.

This is especially helpful when it comes to keeping us alive. It's sad, but most accidents are the result of a lack of awareness and a failure to pay attention to intuition. My guidance often tells me what to do to keep me safe, which is why I pay careful attention to my inner knowing.

I can recall a time when I heard an inner voice tell me to slow down when I was on the freeway traveling at an appropriate speed. This is one of the very few times that the voice of my guidance was loud — to make sure to get my attention. Thankfully, I heeded, because seconds later, a drunk driver careened across the freeway only inches in front of me. Had I not paid attention to my Divine guidance, I would have been broadsided and perhaps killed.

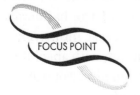

FOCUS POINT

When your body is clogged with foods and thoughts that don't promote serenity and clarity, the waves of information that are available whenever you need them pass right by.

The First Secret to Divine Connection

The first secret to Divine connection is keeping your body clear and healthy, which is what part 2 is all about. You will learn about the second secret of Divine connection in part 3.

Eating the wrong foods might not bring instant death, but given time, it's likely to prove just as deadly as a drunk driver. If you pay attention, your intuition will alert you each time you are tempted to put something harmful in your mouth — provided you understand and care about what junk foods do to your body.

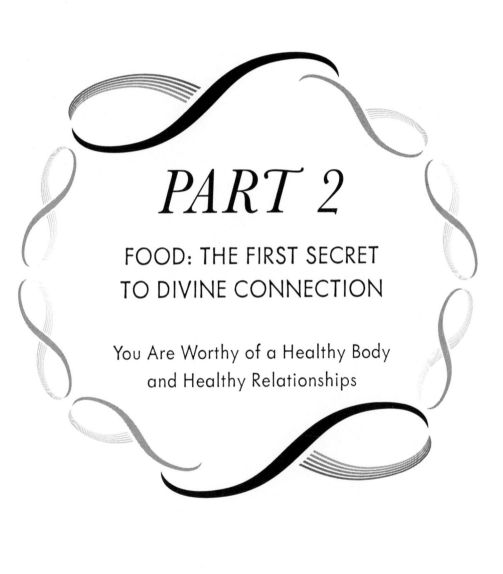

PART 2

FOOD: THE FIRST SECRET
TO DIVINE CONNECTION

You Are Worthy of a Healthy Body
and Healthy Relationships

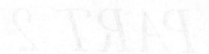

PART 2

CHAPTER 5

REVELATIONS ABOUT THE FOODS YOU EAT

We all have images from our pasts that stay with us. One image that has always stayed with me is from an event that occurred when I was about six years old. Around that time, after WWII, margarine appeared on the market. We were told by the food industry — and the people who allegedly knew what was healthy for us — that butter was bad and margarine was good.

My mother used to purchase the margarine, or "oleo" (short for oleomargarine) as we called it, in one-pound cellophane packets of white squishy fat with a small, round red-orange gelatin capsule wrapped inside on the top. My mother would squeeze the contents of the capsule onto the white mound, and then she would hand it to me to knead the yellow dye into it until it was a buttery yellow. Even at my young age, something about this didn't feel right to me. I adored real butter, but I was repulsed by margarine.

Margarine was made mainly of refined vegetable oil. At that time, we were told that natural fats such as butter, nuts, avocados, and eggs were bad for us and that processed fats such as refined vegetable oils were good. Recent research proves exactly the opposite to be the case. In fact, in *Brain Maker*, Dr. David Perlmutter cites research regarding the explosion of Alzheimer's and other diseases of the brain as being related to not enough healthy natural fats and too much unhealthy processed fats (as cited in chapter 2).

One of the other problems caused by not eating enough healthy fats is that the body will burn carbohydrates rather than fats. When the body burns carbohydrates, which results from eating unhealthy fats and a lot of processed carbohydrates, the fat is stored in the body, which is a major cause of obesity in our culture. When we eat enough healthy fat and fewer processed carbohydrates, the body burns fat, and we lose weight. Unhealthy fats are only one type of food that causes health problems and disconnection from Divine guidance.

The Problem with Grains

People have eaten grains for thousands of years without reacting to them the way they do today. Now even organic grains cause problems. What's different? Part of the answer lies in the way grain is currently harvested. Before the invention of the combine harvester in the mid-1800s, grains were harvested after they sprouted. Unsprouted grains and seeds contain phytic acid, which inhibits digestion and the absorption of some nutrients, particularly minerals. Today grains are harvested before sprouting, which makes a huge difference in how healthy they are. Thus, Sally Fallon writes:

> The process of germination not only produces Vitamin C, but also changes the composition of grains and seeds in numerous beneficial ways. Sprouting increases vitamin B content, especially B2, B5, and B6. Carotene increases dramatically — sometimes eightfold. Even more important, sprouting neutralizes phytic acid, a substance present in the bran of all grains that inhibits the absorption of calcium, magnesium, iron, copper, and zinc; sprouting also neutralizes enzyme inhibitors present in all seeds. These inhibitors can neutralize our own precious enzymes in the digestive tract. Complex sugars responsible for intestinal gas are

broken down during sprouting, and a portion of the starch in grain is transformed into sugar. Sprouting inactivates aflatoxins, potent carcinogens found in grains. Finally, numerous enzymes that help digestion are produced during the germination process.[1]

Fortunately, some companies are starting to sell sprouted seeds and grains, and it's also easy to sprout your own. In addition, according to William Davis, MD, in *Wheat Belly*, practically all wheat, even organic wheat, has been genetically modified, which is why so many people now react to both wheat and the genetically modified form of gluten that's in the wheat, which is often called super gluten.

Original wheat had fourteen chromosomes, but over the years of genetic modifications, it now often contains forty-two chromosomes, which our bodies can't handle. GM wheat, which obviously contains genetically modified gluten, causes major inflammation throughout the body.[2] Of course, bread isn't the only food that contains wheat. Examine most processed and packaged foods, and you will almost always find wheat as one of the ingredients.

I make delicious sourdough bread using half each of sprouted organic rye and sprouted organic einkorn (an ancient form of wheat that has not been genetically modified). I've offered my bread to many gluten-sensitive people. Not one of them has had a negative reaction to the gluten in my bread. Mark Hyman, MD, a well-known functional medicine doctor, states that today's gluten isn't the same as past gluten.[3]

Many are now on the gluten-free bandwagon, but when you look at the ingredients in gluten-free processed foods, you can see that they are anything but healthy. While there are people with celiac disease who need to stay away from gluten and there are some who

---

1.   Sally Fallon, *Nourishing Traditions* (White Plains, Maryland: New Trends Publishing, 2001) p. 112.

2.   William Davis, MD, *Wheat Belly* (Emmaus, Pennsylvania: Rodale Books, 2014) pp. 18–30.

3.   To learn how gluten has changed over the years, see www.mindbodygreen .com/0-14166/is-it-better-to-eat-paleo-or-vegan-dr-mark-hyman-explains.html.

have become gluten-sensitive due to the genetically modified "super gluten," many who seem gluten-sensitive are actually wheat-sensitive and can handle gluten in its natural form, such as in ancient sprouted wheat and other non–genetically modified sprouted grains.

The Nutritional Content of Fruits and Vegetables

In addition to fats and grains, unless you are eating organic, your fruits and vegetables have been sprayed with pesticides and grown on devitalized soil with synthetic fertilizers. Our bodies weren't designed to manage pesticides, and we are being robbed of much-needed minerals because of the devitalized soil. All this lowers not only our immunity but also our vibrancy. The fruits and vegetables grown with GMO seeds (seeds that have been processed with genetically modified organisms) contain GMOs. According to Elizabeth Renter, "Monsanto's GMO corn has been tied to numerous health issues, including weight gain and organ disruption."[4]

Confined Animal Factory Operations

Now we come to the factory farms — confined animal feeding operations, or CAFOs.[5] Not only are the animals on these farms badly abused, but also the beef cattle raised on factory farms, for example, are given antibiotics that you absorb when you eat the meat. These contribute to the dangerous trend of many common antibiotics becoming ineffective. In addition, 80 percent of feedlot cattle are injected with hormones to fatten them up so that they will bring in a greater profit.[6] The cows are typically fed grass that has been sprayed with pesticides, and then they are fed grain, including GMO corn and soy (most corn and soy are genetically modified), during the last few months of their lives, again to fatten them up.

But grain isn't natural to cows. The grain they consume actually changes the composition of their fat, making it unhealthy for

---

4. See "Top 10 Worst GMO Foods for Your GMO Foods List," Natural Society, http://naturalsociety.com/top-10-worst-gmo-foods-list/.
5. For information about CAFOs, go to www.aspca.org/animal-cruelty/factory-farms.
6. Learn about the health issues related to beef and hormones at www.sustainabletable.org/258/hormones.

humans.[7] As with traditional grains, people have eaten meat for thousands of years without encountering the health problems that current factory-farm-produced meats now cause.

Chickens raised in factory farms suffer extreme cruelty.[8] Nonorganic, caged poultry and their eggs are often tainted with pesticides, growth hormones, and antibiotics.[9] Again, all this lowers both your immunity and your energetic vibrancy, resulting in Divine disconnection. The same is true of farmed fish, which are generally contaminated with pesticides, antibiotics, and other chemicals used to fight the diseases and parasites they encounter.[10]

"Nonfood" Milk versus Real Milk

When I was raising my three children in Los Angeles, Alta Dena Dairy delivered organic raw milk and other dairy products right to our door. From the time my babies stopped nursing, they drank raw milk loaded with nutrients not found in pasteurized milk. When raw milk sours (clabbers), it's still safe to drink. No one in my family ever got sick from raw organic milk.

I knew many people who also used raw organic dairy products. Contrary to unsupported public concern about clean, organic, raw dairy products, no one ever got sick. My family took a field trip once to Alta Dena Dairy and saw how clean their facilities were, how healthy the cows were, and how often the milk was tested. The healthy cows didn't need antibiotics to prevent them from getting sick because they ate organic grass, were tested often, and weren't fed grain.

However, as Alta Dena grew bigger, the pasteurized dairy industry became threatened and made up lies about people getting sick from

---

7. For information on why grass-fed beef is more healthful than grain-fed, see the following articles:
   www.mercola.com/beef/health_benefits.htm
   http://chriskresser.com/why-grass-fed-trumps-grain-fed/
   https://authoritynutrition.com/grass-fed-vs-grain-fed-beef/
8. See www.peta.org/issues/animals-used-for-food/factory-farming/chickens.
9. See www.peta.org/issues/animals-used-for-food/factory-farming/chickens /chicken-industry.
10. See http://articles.mercola.com/sites/articles/archive/2013/12/21/9-farmed-fish -facts.aspx

the raw milk.[11] They were successful in forcing Alta Dena to stop selling raw milk; for many years, they had to pasteurize their milk. Now raw milk can be sold in California and a few other states, but in many states, the only way to get it is to purchase a cow share from a local organic dairy, which is how I purchase it in Colorado.

So don't be fooled by the oft-heard claim that raw milk will make you sick. Perpetuated by the pasteurized dairy industry, this claim has no foundation.[12] Quite the contrary, raw milk has been shown to be much safer than pasteurized milk when it originates from a clean dairy where the cows are tested regularly.[13]

I've been drinking raw milk and making yogurt and kefir from it for the past fifty-six years and have never become ill from it. In fact, raw milk has major health benefits.[14] I consider pasteurized dairy to be a nonfood. The pasteurization of milk can cause health problems due to the destruction of valuable beneficial bacteria, enzymes, vitamins, and proteins.[15] Pasteurized milk creates problems in the body, resulting in inflammation and lowered energetic vibrancy.

Sugar

Another nonfood that greatly lowers immunity and vibrancy is sugar.[16] Do you read the labels of processed foods? If you do, you know

---

11. Read about Alta Dena Dairy at http://www.realmilk.com/commentary/vendetta -against-alta-dena-dairy/.
12. Learn more about raw milk here: www.healthfreedoms.org/the-dirty-underbelly -of-the-dairy-industry.
13. You can find valuable information about the overall safety of raw milk at articles. mercola.com/sites/articles/archive/2012/01/14/mark-mcafee-raw-milk-update.aspx.
14. Visit the following sites to learn about the benefits of raw milk:
    http://draxe.com/raw-milk-benefits/
    http://www.drdeborahmd.com/health-benefits-raw-milk
    https://chriskresser.com/raw-milk-reality-benefits-of-raw-milk/
15. Learn about the downsides of pasteurization through the following articles:
    www.westonaprice.org/book-reviews/devil-in-the-milk-by-keith-woodford/
    www.huffingtonpost.com/dr-mercola/dairy-free-avoid-this-pop_b_558447.html
16. Learn about how sugar affects immunity through the following articles:
    www.askdrsears.com/topics/feeding-eating/family-nutrition/sugar/harmful -effects-excess-sugar
    www.ncbi.nlm.nih.gov/pmc/articles/PMC3871217/
    www.healthfreedoms.org/sugar-feeds-cancer-cells-but-it-may-even-create-them/

that most processed foods contain sugar, or they contain ingredients like wheat that turn into sugar in the body.

Sugar and processed foods, as well as artificial sweeteners, feed the deleterious bacteria in the gut and are majorly responsible for creating the imbalance so many suffer from.[17] The brain toxicity caused by sugar and other processed foods results in the lowered vibrancy that makes it difficult to access Divine guidance.

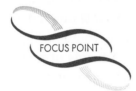

FOCUS POINT

Sugar and other processed foods result in brain toxicity that lowers vibrancy and makes connecting with Divine guidance difficult.

Pink Slime

In 2012, the American public learned about pink slime, an additive that, at that time, was in 70 percent of the meat sold in supermarkets. The slime, which is disinfected with ammonia, used to be sold only to dog food or cooking oil suppliers.[18]

Why does the meat industry use this slime? Because beef will continue to appear pink when it's actually going bad, which increases profit. Is this the kind of meat you really want to eat or feed to your family? Do you want to consume ammonia and parts of the cow that have been exposed to fecal matter?

Many markets stopped selling meat containing pink slime, but unfortunately, it's now making a comeback because beef prices are going through the roof. One way to know whether you are eating pink slime is to look for the terms "finely textured beef" or "textured beef"

---

17. Read about how sugar affects gut health in the following articles and book:
    http://www.globalhealingcenter.com/natural-health/3-ways-sugar-and-artificial
       -sweeteners-affect-gut-health/
    https://iquitsugar.com/it-all-starts-in-your-gut/
    http://www.ncbi.nlm.nih.gov/pmc/articles/PMC1379072/
    John Rudkin, *Pure, White, and Deadly: How Sugar Is Killing Us and What We Can Do to Stop It* (London: Penguin Books, 2013).
18. Read about past uses of pink slime here: www.parenting.blogs.nytimes
    .com/2012/03/09/will-there-be-pink-slime-in-your-childs-school-lunch
    /?scp=1&sq=pink%20slime&st=cse.

on the label.[19] However, the only way to be sure there is no pink slime is to buy organic meat, preferably grass fed.

The food industry has many ways to get away with selling food-like products that are presented as actual food. I abhor the idea of passing off these products as healthy when they are causing major inflammatory conditions in our bodies, and research indicates that chronic inflammation is one of the major causes of illnesses experienced today.[20] If you examine the labels of most packaged foods and research the chemicals listed, you'll discover how much harm is being done to your health by these products that are not only toxic, but also hard to digest — a double whammy in terms of lowering your vibrancy and therefore your ability to connect with Divine guidance.

The Burger

In 2003, Patricia Chopich Reichert (Dr. Erika Chopich's [cocreator of the Inner Bonding process] now deceased sister), worked at Whole Foods Market in Santa Fe, New Mexico, spending much of her time interviewing prospective employees and training new hires. The six-week training program included hands-on experience as well as many classes. Employees learned to read labels and discuss the pros and cons of food additives and chemicals. Someone asked whether it's true that undertakers use less embalming fluid these days due to the amount of preservatives in our food.

Patricia walked to a closet and removed a McDonald's bag. Seated at the table, she removed a second bag that was all but shredded from use and age. From the inner bag, she removed a wrapped single plain burger and a small bag of fries that were in perfect-looking condition. The smell of rancid, saturated grease permeated the air as she explained, "This has never been refrigerated. The bag has been in the closet since the day these items were purchased. This burger just looks cold, doesn't it? There is no mold on the fries. No insects

---

19. Learn more about how to avoid pink slime here: http://www.clarkhoward.com /how-to-know-if-youre-eating-pink-slime.
20. Amy Myers, MD, *The Autoimmune Solution* (San Francisco: HarperOne, 2017) pp. 11, 16, 93–94, and 183.

are here. No rodent has ever investigated. Clearly, the bag has deteriorated more than the food. The receipt has faded so that you can barely read it, but I can tell you that the date says January 12, 2000. Yes, these items are over three years old!"

Have you ever tried to connect with your Divine guidance after eating at McDonald's or another fast-food place? It likely wouldn't have occurred to you if you connected before eating, because you would not have chosen to eat junky fast food in the first place. I'm one of the few people I know who has never eaten at McDonald's! I have never regretted it.

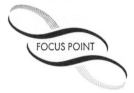

FOCUS POINT

Try connecting to your Divine guidance when you have the urge to eat fast food. You will likely be guided in another direction.

Health Starts in the Gut

Today, we are increasingly aware of how so many of our health issues come down to an imbalance of healthy versus unhealthy gut bacteria because of the foods we eat, the pharmaceuticals we use, and the stress we experience. With this in mind, I would like to review the roots of the problem that cause so much illness, low vibrancy, and disconnection from your Divine guidance. They are as follows:

Processed foods. These are precisely what the term implies — foods altered from their natural state. Because they have been refined, many of the nutrients the body needs are absent. Often, unhealthy food-like products have been added, such as high fructose corn syrup (HFCS), GMOs, trans fats, preservatives, coloring, and so on. All cause inflammation and destroy beneficial flora.

Sugared food-like products. Sugar and sugar-like products not only destroy beneficial bacteria but also feed toxic bacteria. This is why the more we eat sugar, HFCS, and white refined products that turn into sugar in the body, the more we crave these things. As toxic bacteria proliferate, they demand more and more sugar to flourish. The more they flourish, the more they create toxins that inflame our organs and our brains, causing physical and mental illness and leading to spiritual disconnection.

Antibiotics, other drugs, and synthetic supplements. Antibiotics destroy harmful bacteria, and they kill beneficial bacteria. This leaves the gut vulnerable to more harmful bacteria unless the beneficial bacteria are replaced with probiotic supplements together with prebiotic and probiotic foods. Many prescription and over-the-counter drugs also destroy beneficial bacteria. Surprisingly, so do most synthetic vitamins and minerals, which are often manufactured by drug companies. Supplements need to be whole-food based to be effective and not destroy our beneficial gut bacteria.[21]

Factory-farmed meat, poultry, fish, and dairy. These products from CAFOs contain antibiotics and hormones given to the animals plus pesticides that are in their feed. This destroys beneficial bacteria. In addition, when cows are fed grain instead of grass, their fat no longer contains many of the nutrients beneficial for our guts, organs, and brains.

Chlorinated water. Chlorine is as hard on our gut as antibiotics, and we are adversely affected by both drinking and showering in unfiltered chlorinated water.[22]

Household cleaning products and cosmetics. Even cleaning products, antibacterial soaps, toothpaste, and other everyday products can create an imbalance in the gut because of the chemicals they contain.[23]

Being "too clean." Our focus on cleanliness, including antibiotic soaps, strip the good bacteria from our hands, which has led to less beneficial bacteria in the gut. In addition, since most people no longer grow their own food, they are not getting their hands in the dirt or eating fruits and vegetables right from the garden. Unwashed

---

21. Brian R. Clement, PhD, *Supplements Exposed* (Wayne, New Jersey: New Page Books, 2009) pp. 43–44.

22. Learn more about the effects of chlorine here:
    http://www.thecandidadiet.com/chlorine-immune-system.htm
    http://www.everydayhealth.com/columns/therese-borchard-sanity-break/strange-links-among-chlorine-candida-depression/
    http://www.motherjones.com/environment/2014/07/case-against-chlorinated-tap-water

23. Natasha Campbell-McBride, *Gut and Psychology Syndrome* (Norfolk, UK: MedInform Publishing, 2010).

garden-fresh produce is filled with beneficial bacteria that we now rarely eat. Each tablespoon of healthy soil contains more beneficial bacteria than there are people on the planet! We need to get our hands in more good dirt![24]

From this list, you can readily see why most people are suffering from a grave imbalance in their gut flora. If you want to connect with your spiritual guidance, you need to do healing work to reduce inflammation and restore the natural balance.

24. Learn about healthy soil microbes at http://extension.oregonstate.edu/gardening /secret-life-soil-0.

CHAPTER 6

THE GUT-BRAIN-SPIRIT CONNECTION

For the first twenty-two years of my life, I was unaware that it's hard for our bodies not only to deal with processed foods but also to eliminate some of the chemicals used in them, which accumulate in our bodies — especially in our fat — and add to our toxic load. I had been a sickly child, and because I lacked information and ate a lot of sugar, I was a sickly young woman. I hated being so.

When I turned twenty-two and found I lacked the energy I wanted to have, I began studying everything I could get my hands on concerning health and nutrition and markedly improved my diet. As I began eating as close to nature as possible, my health improved dramatically. Clearly I was on the right track.

As Gerard E. Mullin, MD, (associate professor of medicine at John Hopkins University School of Medicine) comments, "One of the most obvious and profound consistencies among traditional diets like the MedDiet and the Baltic Sea diet is the focus on real, whole, healing foods, not the processed junk food that dominates the modern Western diet. More than any of the other healthy elements of traditional eating, this may be the key differentiating factor."[1]

Before doing the gut-brain research, I didn't understand why the way I was eating made such a difference in my ability to connect with Divine guidance. I knew that things like sugar, pesticides, preservatives, and processed foods lowered my vibrancy, making it much harder for me to connect, but I never understood the underlying dynamics regarding this.

Recent research suggests that creating a healthy and balanced microbiome — a healthy balance of gut flora — is essential for health and vibrancy. Current research indicates that gut dysbiosis (an imbalanced gut) is a major contributor to many illnesses.[2]

It is now becoming common knowledge that health starts in the gut, and the health of the gut flora is destroyed by sugar, wheat, and processed foods; antibiotics and other drugs; and chlorinated water, household cleaning chemicals, and airborne toxins. Gut imbalance is also a major factor in anxiety and depression. Toxicity in the gut creates toxicity in the brain.[3]

While it might be hard to understand that what goes on in the gut has a huge effect on the brain, we have only to remember what happens when we drink alcohol. The alcohol goes into the gut and then very quickly affects your brain.

Toxicity in the gut causes you to not be able to raise your frequency high enough to connect with Divine guidance. Because of the connection between the gut and the brain, you will have a hard time connecting with your guidance if your gut and your brain are toxic.

People try many different ways to connect with their guidance but still can't consistently connect. You might even be "eating well" and still be unable to connect. What you call eating well and what current research calls eating well may be two entirely different things.

---

1. Gerard E. Mullin, MD, *The Gut Balance Revolution* (Emmaus, Pennsylvania: Rodale Press, Inc., 2017) p. 148.
2. Dr. David Perlmutter, *Brain Maker* (Boston: Little, Brown and Company, 2015) pp. 8–11, 20, and 37–39.
3. Dr. David Perlmutter, *Brain Maker* (Boston: Little, Brown and Company, 2015) pp. 81–87.

And while what you eat has a huge effect on your vibrancy, so do your thoughts and actions.

If you eat extremely well but you indulge in junk thoughts (which we will address in part 3), you will greatly limit your ability to connect with Divine guidance. If you raise your consciousness and stop your junk thoughts but continue to eat junk foods, Divine connection will likely still elude you. Learning about how the gut affects the brain has helped me understand why I have an easy time connecting with my Divine guidance.

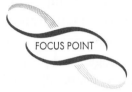

FOCUS POINT

Toxicity in the gut results in toxicity in the brain, creating a barrier to your Divine guidance.

How the Gut Can Become Out of Balance Early in Life

A baby is born with a sterile gut. Babies get their first dose of specific and beneficial gut flora as they come through the birth canal because, in a healthy woman, the birth canal is full of beneficial bacteria. However, if the mother is not healthy — as my mother wasn't due to intense antibiotics from a ruptured appendix — then the baby receives opportunistic, unhealthy bacteria. If the baby is born via C-section, he or she also misses out on the healthy gut flora.

The next dose of specific and hopefully healthy bacteria comes to a baby through the mother's milk. Again, if the mother is unhealthy, then the baby receives unhealthy bacteria. If the mother doesn't breastfeed, the baby doesn't receive the beneficial bacteria. If the baby is fed formula with soy or preservatives, any good bacteria are quickly destroyed and can be further destroyed by antibiotics, drugs, chlorinated water, and processed foods. This leaves the child open to many physical and emotional problems.

It is evident from current research that a problem with gut bacteria — when the unhealthy bacteria overrun the healthy bacteria — may not only create brain symptoms such as autism, schizophrenia, ADD, ADHD, bipolar disorder, OCD, Asperger's, learning disabilities, and so on, but also digestive disorders, colic in babies, Crohn's disease, asthma, allergies, food intolerances, and eventually diabetes, auto-immune diseases, heart disease, and cancer.[4] Gut dysbiosis may very well be one of the major causes of many illnesses, along with numerous viruses such as the Epstein Barr Virus (EBV), that are covertly affecting our health, and it's likely that more research will prove this.[5]

Gaining an understanding of how to heal the gut and how to render viruses inactive is vital for all of us. A baby whose immune system is compromised in these ways and who receives many rounds of antibiotics for ear and throat infections could become vulnerable to autism. Much research is being done on the relationship between the gut and autism.[6] Twenty years ago, 1 in 20,000 children were diagnosed with autism; now it's 1 in 45. Unhealthy parents, C-sections, fewer women breastfeeding, antibiotics, sugar and processed foods, environmental chemicals, and chlorinated water all contribute to the imbalance of flora in the intestines. They also contribute to the proliferation of disease and viruses.

Is it any wonder that there is a dumbing down going on in our society? Unfortunately, this dumbing down leads to disconnection from ourselves and our Divine guidance, which makes it easier for us to be controlled through the plethora of TV commercials and fake news. If we can't tap into our inner knowing and access the truth, we can be easily controlled by the authorities and the powers that be.

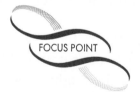

FOCUS POINT

When we can't tap into our inner knowing and access the truth, others can easily control us.

4. Dr. Natasha Campbell-McBride, *Gut and Psychology Syndrome* (MedInform Publishing, 2004) pp. 5–7.; Dr. David Perlmutter, *Brain Maker* (Boston: Little, Brown and Company, 2015) pp. 5–6 and 47; and Dr. Gerald Mullins, *Gut Balance Revolution* (Emmaus, Pennsylvania: Rodale Press, 2015) pp. 18–21, and 88.

5. Dr. Amy Myers, *The Autoimmune Solution (San Francisco:* HarperOne, 2015) pp. 16, 150–155, and 162–163, and Anthony William, *Medical Medium* (Carlsbad: Hay House, Inc., 2015) pp. 39–61.

6. See the following websites for information on the gut-autism research currently under way: https://link.springer.com/article/10.1007/s11920-012-0337-0, https://www.sciencedaily.com/releases/2017/06/170619101834.htm, and http://www.tandfonline.com/doi/abs/10.3402/mehd.v23i0.19260.

It is unrealistic to expect that you will have enough vibrancy to access your Divine guidance when your brain is toxic. Since I have, for most of my life, been eating almost exactly the way much current research recommends, I now understand a major reason why it's so easy for me to access my guidance.

As I've stated, there is no one right way of eating that works for everyone. You need to discover whether a particular diet — the Medi-Diet, the Paleo Diet, a raw diet — or being a vegan or vegetarian is what works best for you. There are numerous ways of creating a healthy gut and rendering viruses inactive, and to support your ability to connect with Divine guidance, you need to educate yourself regarding what works for you so that a toxic brain doesn't prevent your connection. I will help you determine how you can eat to most support your vibrancy and ability to connect with your Divine guidance.

Anxiety and Depression: Your Gut and Your Gut Feelings

When people are depressed, psychiatrists frequently don't know how to help them. Lacking any real understanding of the nature of depression, they turn to a pharmaceutical that (at least for a time) serves as a crutch for lifting their patient's spirits. The problem is that the chemicals administered mask the problem instead of address the cause and, as you will see, have primarily a placebo effect.

June 18, 2015, the day after the murder of nine members of an African Methodist Episcopal congregation in Charleston by Dylann Roof, President Barack Obama stood righteous, angry, but powerless as he sought to respond to yet another mass killing by a gunman. "I've had to make statements like this too many times," he lamented, referring to the fourteen mass killings that occurred during his presidency.[7]

Why is America a land of so many mass shootings? Researchers have identified a common thread that runs through not only almost every mass shooting but also many cases of isolated shootings and suicides. This thread is that "all of the perpetrators were either actively taking powerful psychotropic drugs or had been at some point in the

---

7. Read the article at www.theatlantic.com/politics/archive/2015/06/president -obama-on-charleston-shooting-ive-had-to-make-statements-like-this-too-many -times/453312/.

immediate past before they committed their crimes."[8] This is a stunning revelation, and it comes not from just a single study but from "multiple credible scientific studies going back more than a decade."

Even more alarming is the fact that "internal documents from certain pharmaceutical companies that suppressed the information show that SSRI drugs (selective serotonin re-uptake inhibitors) have well known, but unreported side effects, including but not limited to suicide and other violent behavior."

Dylann Roof was taking a drug that has been linked to sudden outbursts of violence, "fitting the pattern of innumerable other mass shooters who were on or had recently come off pharmaceutical drugs linked to aggression." Stephen Paddock, the Las Vegas shooter, "was prescribed an anti-anxiety drug in June that can lead to aggressive behavior."[9]

SSRIs don't cure the depression for which they are prescribed; they only mask it. The fact is that these drugs are a substitute for a cure and are used only because psychiatrists don't understand the real causes of depression and therefore don't know what else to do for the severely depressed.

Depression doesn't come out of nowhere. I've discovered three major causes of depression:

- unresolved trauma/posttraumatic stress disorder
- self-abandonment
- a toxic gut, resulting in a toxic brain

I will be addressing the first two causes in the part 3. It's important not to confuse depression with the sadness and grief from life's painful experiences. Current painful experiences, such as the loss of a loved one; natural disasters; physical or emotional trauma; frightening financial situations; marital and family challenges; a bully boss; and violent situations such as rape, beatings, theft, and war cause

---

8.   Read about this revelation at the following websites:
     www.ammoland.com/2013/04/every-mass-shooting-in-the-last-20-years-shares
     -psychotropic-drugs/#axzz4zt0Yqrzb
     www.cchrflorida.org/antidepressants-are-a-prescription-for-mass-shootings/
     www.naturalnews.com/039752_mass_shootings_psychiatric_drugs_antidepressants
9.   See the article explaining the shooter's prescription here: www.reviewjournal.com
     /local/the-strip/las-vegas-strip-shooter-prescribed-anti-anxiety-drug-in-june/.

much sadness, sorrow, grief, heartbreak, and feelings of helplessness. They always take considerable time to heal. These feelings are normal and should not be avoided in any way or suppressed with medication.

However, when you have never learned how to manage these painful life feelings and you then abandon yourself in the face of current challenging situations, you might also feel depressed. When the distress you experience is accompanied by self-abandonment, things can go awry. Life calls forth our capacity for resilience, which enables us to pass through painful times and come out the other side strengthened. However, if you haven't learned how to lovingly manage painful times, you can easily sink into depression.

The last thing people need when going through a painful time is to deny the pain, burying it. Instead, they need the Divine support that helps them draw on their inner resources so that they can face these times with resilience and equanimity.

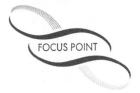

FOCUS POINT

In painful times, do not deny or bury your pain. Instead, draw on your inner resources to face those times with resilience and equanimity.

It was not that long ago when we thought having a "stiff upper lip" was the way people got through tough times. Today we have swung to the other extreme, whereby we don't want anyone to suffer any degree of emotional discomfort and consequently drug them up with antidepressants to numb their pain. Neither approach is healthy. Neither promotes long-term well-being.

What prevents some of us from tapping into our resilience when life is distressing? Why can one person go through the grieving process and come out strengthened and another survives from day to day only with the deadening effect of psychotropic drugs? One reason is that many people have never learned how to lovingly manage their feelings.[10] However, as I stated above, there is also a physical cause for the lack of resilience.

---

10. To begin to learn how to do this, take the free Inner Bonding course at http://www.innerbonding.com/welcome.

As we explored earlier in this chapter, new research is revealing how an imbalance of intestinal flora can result in a toxic state that adversely affects the brain, often resulting in anxiety and depression. To illustrate how this works, I'll use my former sugar addiction. On a physical level, a sugar addiction revolves around what's going on in the digestive system. If we have more beneficial intestinal flora than harmful flora, we have a healthy gut and likely won't crave sugar.

When I was young, my parents didn't have access to the knowledge that clean, natural, organic foods nurture beneficial gut bacteria and that sugar and processed food-like products promote inflammation and the proliferation of microorganisms that are detrimental to us. So they did not understand that I had a sugar craving, which is one reason I was a sickly child. The other main reason was that, as I previously stated, my mother was given heavy antibiotics before I was born, so I likely started life with an unhealthy gut. When we indulge in sugary foods, along with other nonfoods on the shelves of our supermarkets, we stress the body, overloading it with toxins to the point that our systems are unable to eliminate them in the normal way.

When we add to this state of toxicity the almost constant stress so many of us are under (which produces its own toxic effects on body chemistry) and at the same time deprive ourselves of purifying elements — such as exercise, exposure to sunshine (to promote the uptake of the hormone we commonly refer to as vitamin D and other benefits of being outside, such as the high frequency of nature), adequate sleep, water that hasn't been contaminated with chemicals (such as fluoride and chlorine), and a supply of macronutrients and micronutrients from wholesome organic fruits and vegetables — it's not difficult to see how the gut microbiota can end up way out of whack.

As I have stated, the source of much illness is inflammation caused by sugar, super gluten, unsprouted grains, factory-farmed meats and produce, pasteurized milk and other pasteurized dairy, and the unhealthy processed fats from seed and nut oils (soybean, cottonseed, canola, and the like), resulting in an imbalanced gut microbiome.[11] Contrary to what we were previously told, we need the

---

11. Dr. Amy Myers, *The Autoimmune Solution* (San Francisco: HarperOne, 2015) pp. 11, 16, 93–94, and 183.

natural healthy fats from avocado, olive, and coconut oils, as well as other natural fats. (As I cited earlier, one of the causes of Alzheimer's is a lack of healthy fats.[12])

An impaired microbiome delivers toxins directly to the brain through the vagus nerve, which can result in anxiety, depression, and many other disorders.[13] Medication prescribed to ease these conditions does just the opposite, intensifying the toxicity and thereby exacerbating the condition. As Dr. Irving Kirsch reveals, antidepressants have a mostly placebo effect, and despite their much-touted and frequently prescribed status, they are simply not as effective as psychotherapy.[14]

Would it surprise you to hear that the supposed imbalance in the brain that antidepressants are intended to address is something the drug companies made up? The brain doesn't need drugs to operate efficiently. Rather, it's the imbalance in the gut that causes brain toxicity.[15]

Through current research, we are increasingly coming to see just how extensively the microbiota that populate our gastrointestinal tract depend on the quality of our dietary choices for their ability to regulate the immune system. The types of carbohydrates, fiber, protein, and fats we ingest alter the composition of the gut microbiota. This in turn modifies how our food is processed and ultimately modulates our immunity and hence our vibrancy.

Few of us have any awareness of just how many aspects of our modern society destroy the healthy bacteria native to the human digestive system, leaving us not only physically but also emotionally vulnerable to the ravages of unhealthy bacteria, as well as to the various viruses that make their home in our bodies. So we see that research is revealing

12. Dr. David Perlmutter, *Brain Maker* (Boston: Little, Brown and Company, 2015) pp. 46 and 60.
13. Learn more about gut-brain toxicity here: https://www.ncbi.nlm.nih.gov /pubmed/24997031.
14. Dr. Irving Kirsch, *The Emperor's New Drugs: Exploding the Antidepressant Myth* (Random House, 2009) pp. 101–148, and 163. Also see YouTube video https:// www.youtube.com/watch?v=wNLoiKo8z3Y&t=3s.
15. Dr. David Perlmutter, *Brain Maker* (Boston: Little, Brown and Company, 2015) pp. 81–87.

the direct connection between the gut and the brain and thus how junk foods create toxicity in the gut that goes to the brain.

In a nutshell, when the gut microbiome becomes sufficiently deranged, we too can become deranged. When you ask people at random about depression, they tend to say something similar to, "It's a chemical imbalance in the brain." Dr. David Perlmutter refutes this, asserting, "Two decades of scientific literature highlight the role of inflammation in mental illness, from depression to schizophrenia..."[16] He explains that our gut's microbes control the production of inflammatory chemicals in the body, which in turn become factors that affect our mental health. He adds, "The connection between depression and the gut is not new information."[17]

By learning how to create a healthy gut, we humans can heal ourselves of much of our dysfunction without resorting to drugs to cover up the problem. Clearly, understanding and correcting the problems with our gut microbiota has implications for the well-being of our entire planet — indeed, for our ongoing evolution as a species. It's important to point out that in this book, "gut" refers not only to our microbiota but also to what we commonly refer to as our gut feelings. This is significant, because it's no accident that we associate feelings with the gut.

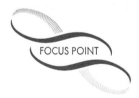

FOCUS POINT

When we create and maintain a healthy gut, we improve our lives and help the planet.

We ought to be able to trust our gut, since the gut is intended to function as an extension of the brain, in a sense acting as a brain all of its own. When the gut is in disorder, our gut feelings are going to be

16. Dr. David Perlmutter, *Brain Maker* (Boston: Little, Brown and Company, 2015) p. 75.
17. Bested AC, Logan AC, Selhub EM. "Intestinal Microbiota, Probiotics and Mental Health: From Metchnikoff to Modern Advances: Part II — Contemporary Contextual Research," *Gut Pathogens*, vol. 5, no. 1 (March 16, 2013); 3, doi: 101186;1757-4749-5-3.

in disarray and therefore likely to mislead us — which is how we end up with mass murders such as the one carried out by Dylann Roof.

Learn to Have Faith over Fear

Old programming can become lodged in both the brain and the gut brain with the result that fear instead of faith often rules us. When challenged to embark on something new, how many people experience a gut reaction from which they conclude that they shouldn't follow what their souls are urging?

When the gut microbiome is in a healthy balance, the fear that's a key element of many of our gut feelings no longer limits us by keeping us stuck in our old, often dysfunctional ways. The gut and the brain unite, along with the heart, so that head, heart, and gut pilot us through life, keeping our spirits intact even in the most painful circumstances life may throw at us. This is the source of the resilience of which we have been speaking, which is the true antidote to depression.

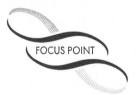

FOCUS POINT

When the gut and the brain unite, along with the heart, so that head, heart, and gut pilot us through life, our spirit remains intact even in the most painful circumstances.

Since psychotropic drugs can't cure depression, no small number of psychotherapists, counselors, coaches, social workers, and others in the helping professions find themselves just as stumped when faced with a deeply depressed person — despite the fact that psychotherapy has been shown to be more effective than antidepressants. I was trained as a traditional psychotherapist and practiced traditionally for seventeen years, but I was unhappy with the results. I also worked with many psychotherapists and many different modalities on my own issues, but I was not happy with the result I was getting personally either.

Not one of the many therapists I worked with told me that I was responsible for lovingly learning from and managing my own feelings. Nor did they have any idea how to help me learn to love myself, and not one explained that this is exceedingly difficult to pull off if we lack a Divine connection. Looking back, I'm amazed at that!

I began seeking a process that would work more deeply and also more quickly than what I was doing. My prayer was answered when, more than thirty-four years ago, I met Dr. Erika Chopich, and Spirit brought us the Inner Bonding process. It became clear to me that a spiritual connection is essential to psychological well-being, and maintaining this connection requires a clear brain.

Here is where healing your gut comes into the picture. As I've said, you will have a hard time connecting with Divine guidance if your brain is awash with toxicity. When people embark on a spiritual path, I find they tend to emphasize heart over head, often to the point that the head is seen as the villain. This is not only unbalanced but also shortsighted. We were given both head and heart, and both are essential to chart a meaningful course through life.

The problem with how the head has so often misled us is that it hasn't been the clear, aware, conscious instrument that it's capable of being. It's been clouded with extraneous thought, much of it driven by emotional reactivity. A clear head goes hand in hand with a quiet mind, not one that's turbulent with conflicting thoughts as we debate ad nauseam even minutiae that don't matter at all.

If you've a problem with your head chattering away all the time, clarity will escape you. For clarity to arise, the mind needs to become still so that awareness becomes its modus operandi. One of the most powerful tools for accomplishing this is to adopt the diet that's right for you as well as to learn to value your soul, which you can do only through your Divine connection.

CHAPTER 7

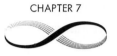

DETERMINE WHAT MOTIVATES YOU TO LIVE WELL

Just as the right motivation is needed if we are to maintain a healthy schedule of exercise, I've discovered two completely different reasons people choose to eat well. These two motivating factors are exact opposites — fear and love.

Some people eat well purely out of fear of becoming sick, growing old and decrepit, or getting fat. With some, the fear is intense enough that they never return to eating badly. Others are motivated by fear for a time but then relapse, and they might cycle through eating well and relapse again and again. Over the long haul, fear tends to be a poor motivator. Its effectiveness is short term and, for many of us, not sustainable.

Others eat well because they love themselves enough to create a healthy temple to house their wonderful souls. When loving yourself is your highest priority, eating well becomes relatively easy.

I became motivated to eat well not only because I was tired of being sick but also because I wanted to be strong and healthy in my older years. I didn't want to eat healthily just to avoid a heart attack or cancer. I wanted to eat well so that I could live life to the fullest. Now, fifty-six years after making this life-changing decision to eat all organic and listen to what my body truly needs, I enjoy excellent health, tons of energy, and the high vibrancy that allows me to stay connected with my Divine guidance.

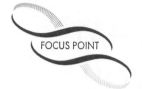

FOCUS POINT

When loving yourself is your highest priority, eating well becomes relatively easy.

At one of my five-day intensives, a discussion arose concerning how food affects our frequency. I shared with the group that I could not maintain a high level of frequency when I ate junk food and that even a small amount would lower my sensation of aliveness and my ability to connect with my Divine source.

One of the participants at the intensive confessed that she had always struggled with being motivated to eat well, which in her case meant that she also struggled with her weight. Now, for the first time, she understood why it is essential to eat well. She finally felt motivated by a desire to achieve a high level of vibrancy, which in turn would allow her to establish a clear channel for her Divine source to guide her.

It's not that many of us aren't aware, at least on a surface level. After all, courtesy of the media, we are bombarded with how sugar, soft drinks, some kinds of fats, and fried foods are bad for us. There's even a growing awareness that devitalized foods (foods that need to be enriched, packaged, and processed), pesticide-laden foods, and factory-farmed foods cause and contribute to illness. Given the ubiquity of information, what causes many of us to ignore the research and go right on eating poorly?

Your wounded ego will often suggest you are making a mistake when you give up a cherished addiction, particularly a food addiction. It has many ways of rationalizing why you should hang on to your addictions, especially as you start to feel the emotional or physical withdrawal symptoms. You might tell yourself something like the following:

• "Life is too short to give up these pleasures. What's the point?

Why not just enjoy it while I can? So what if I cut a few years off my life? It's worth it."

- "Maybe this isn't the right day to start eating differently. I really want that doughnut. I'll start eating well tomorrow. One more day of eating junk won't hurt me."

- "Life just isn't worth living without cigarettes. I love smoking so much. Not everybody who smokes gets lung cancer, so why go through this hell? Anyway, the stress of not smoking is worse for me than the cigarettes."

If you fall for these or other rationalizations, giving into your wounded ego, you will be handing yourself a pacifier rather than love. You will force yourself to be satisfied with the illusion of nurturing rather than the true joy and sense of well-being that comes from bringing through Divine love and taking loving action for yourself. I explored this issue with some of my clients. This is what they revealed, followed by comments I have added (in italics):

- "I don't believe it matters. My parents didn't eat well, and they lived long lives." *When I asked them whether their parents lived healthy, fit, pain-free, long lives, they answered no.*

- "I don't feel any different when I eat junk than when I eat well, so I don't think it's worth the added expense and trouble." *In the short term, perhaps the person isn't aware of the difference, but time will reveal just how great the difference is.*

- "In exchange for a few years off my life, it's worth it to enjoy eating the things I enjoy." *This ignores the fact that many of people's later years, even though shortened, are likely to be spent in illness and perhaps considerable pain, quite apart from the spiritual disconnection the individual experiences.*

Most people will say that they really want to be healthy and spiritually connected. But what are you willing to do to be healthy and attain the vibrancy necessary for Divine connection? Perhaps even more important, what are you ready to no longer do? How willing are you to investigate for yourself what makes for healthy, vibrant living and Divine connection instead of going along with what others say?

Is it more important to eat fast food or packaged and processed food than to take the time to cook healthy meals with healthy ingredients? Would you rather spend money on clothes, restaurants, and vacations than on healthy food?

Do you prefer to sleep in, watch TV, play video games, gamble, work all hours, talk on the phone, and text or engage in other addictive activities than to exercise? Is resorting to pharmaceuticals to handle your anxiety, depression, or insomnia preferable to learning how to lovingly manage pain and rid your life of the poor habits and toxic elements that cause these problems? Do you turn to substances for relief rather than learn how to take responsibility for your feelings?

Are you content to act out addictively with alcohol, cigarettes, sugar, caffeine, and so forth rather than learn to take loving care of yourself? How about taking the time to nurture a sense of inner peace through emotional and spiritual practices such as meditation, journaling, and the self-healing Inner Bonding process that you will learn in the next section?

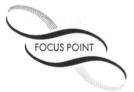

FOCUS POINT

What are you willing to do to be healthy and attain the vibrancy necessary for Divine connection? Perhaps even more important, what are you ready to no longer do?

It's easy to be one of the group — eating like everyone else, drinking like everyone else, or relying on pharmaceuticals — rather than to support your health and vitality. But when you do so, how do you rationalize your unhealthy choices?

Maybe you tell yourself you don't have time to eat well or exercise. Or perhaps you resort to the dubious argument that so-and-so "smoked his whole life and never got lung cancer." Some of us tell ourselves because we're still young, we don't need to worry about our health for a long time to come. Others argue that we're not giving up sweets because they are one of the few rewards we get to enjoy.

The questions to ask yourself are these: "How do I want to live my later years? Do I want to be vital, clearheaded, and energetic? Or am I resigned to suffering from arthritis or some other autoimmune disease, getting cancer, heart disease, or some other degenerative condition such as diabetes?"

Exercise Supports Divine Connection

So far I've focused on diet as we look at the physical aspects of health. But eating a healthy diet alone is not sufficient for maintaining vibrancy. Frequent movement of the body must be included in the picture — not just sitting at a desk all day, but standing, taking plenty of steps, and engaging in some kind of exercise.

Are you aware that lack of exercise is responsible for as many deaths as smoking and obesity?[1] The body requires exercise to stay healthy, which means that failing to make sufficient exercise a priority constitutes a form of self-abandonment. Do you have a regular exercise routine, or are you resistant to exercise? And if you don't exercise, why not? What causes you to abandon yourself in this way?

I've listened to client after client trot out every excuse for not exercising:

- "It's boring."
- "I don't have time."
- "If I get up early enough to exercise, I don't get enough sleep."
- "After working all day, I'm too tired."
- "I don't believe it's that important."

Like good nutrition, exercise needs to be pleasurable if you're going to stick with it. If it feels like a tedious chore, you'll resist it and end up neglecting it. You'll build it into your schedule only if you love it. In fact, when it's something you enjoy, you look forward to it and find the time for it, as I can personally attest.

The challenge is to discover what physical activity you like so

---

1. Physical inactivity causes one in ten deaths worldwide according to a series of studies released in the British medical journal *The Lancet*, putting it on par with the dangers of smoking and obesity. The results also suggest that public health officials treat this situation as a pandemic. Harvard researchers say inactivity caused an increase in deaths from coronary heart disease, type 2 diabetes, and breast and colon cancers, causing more than 5.3 million deaths in 2008 worldwide (http://www.cnn.com/2012/07/18/health/physical-inactivity-deaths /index.html?hpt=hp_bn12).

much that it becomes an essential part of your day or at least something you participate in several times a week over your lifetime. Do you like to dance, play tennis, or shoot baskets? Do you enjoy yoga, jogging, walks in nature, or hiking? Maybe you prefer to work out at a gym, take an aerobics class, or engage in Pilates. There's the option of walking or running on a treadmill while watching TV or listening to a book, or you might prefer reading on an exercise bike.

Exercising in nature has added benefits because the cells of the body are bathed in the high frequency of nature whenever we are outside. My parents, who took fairly good care of themselves physically, both walked and danced as their forms of exercise, so it's no surprise that walking and dancing are favorites with me. To set the tone for my day, I spend time in nature each morning by walking up and down hills. For me, it's also a good time to pray, expressing what's on my mind and in my heart. I use it to further my Inner Bonding process, speaking out loud as I walk. It's rare for me to miss my walk because it's something I love to do and have been doing for many years.

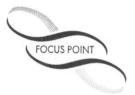

FOCUS POINT

The challenge is to discover what physical activity you like so much that it becomes an essential part of your day or at least something you participate in several times a week over your lifetime.

Horseback riding is a sport I took up as a child, developed as an adolescent, and still enjoy as an older adult. I also take time to throw pots on my pottery wheel. Not only is it beneficial for my hands, wrists, arms, and core, but I love potting and have potted on and off all my adult life.

Then there's my garden. I absolutely relish working in my garden, growing yummy organic fruits and veggies. Years before I had the land for my garden, my father had a large organic garden, which is what I believe kept my parents healthy in their later years. When I adopted a healthy organic lifestyle, my father followed suit with his wonderful organic garden in Santa Monica, California. I loved visiting my parents to "shop" in his garden!

There were a couple of years when I worked out at a gym. I liked it but didn't love it. I tried it again a few years ago and found it just didn't do it for me. I didn't like exercising indoors, and it made my body hurt — a sure sign it wasn't right for me. I've also tried yoga on and off, which I think is a great form of exercise, but it doesn't work well for my body.

I was intrigued by research into the lives of those who live to be a great age. There are five places around the world where people generally live to be over 100. It turns out these long-lived people move naturally. As Dan Buettner discovered, "The world's longest-lived people don't pump iron or run marathons. Instead their environments nudge them into moving without thinking about it."[2]

Try some ways to move in your everyday environment. It's certainly the easiest way to obtain the exercise you need. But don't imagine that the recommended amount of exercise will solve a weight problem. More than 700 studies show that changing your diet is far more effective. As *Science Daily* reported, "Surprisingly, total weight gain in every country was greater among participants who met the physical activity guidelines. For example, American men who met the guidelines gained a half pound per year, while American men who did not meet the guideline lost 0.6 pounds."[3] Exercise tends to increase our hunger, upping our calorie intake in the course of the day. To eat right for our bodies is essential for weight control.

Genes and Hormones Are Also About Food and Mood

In recent decades, there has been much emphasis on the role of genes in promoting health and triggering disease. Often in the shadow is the issue of what activates the genes, which in many instances can be traced to environmental factors. Just how a gene expresses can depend on both the internal environment and the world around us. We are now realizing that the vitality of the food we consume has a

2. See the following websites for Dan Buettner's comments about activities people in blue zones participate in: https://www.forbes.com/sites/devinthorpe /2014/10/08/author-with-longevity-secrets-seeks-to-apply-lessons-to-millions /#5a6f1ffa5ab1 and http://www.youmustbetrippin.com/travel-tips/the-power -9-live-longer-and-happier/

3. *Science Daily*, Loyola University Health Study. February 3, 2017. (https://www .sciencedaily.com/releases/2017/02/170203163857.htm).

powerful effect on epigenetic expression, activating or suppressing genes to either our benefit or detriment.

We are all subject to our genes, the impact of environmental factors, the potential for accidents, and the long-lasting effects of trauma. Why would we want to compound these negatives by neglecting what we have the power to affect positively?

Demonstrating how the immune system is influenced by our diet, the field of psychoneuroimmunology draws on the long-recognized unity of the human. We understand that whether our neurotransmitters and hormones function correctly is tied directly to our nutritional intake — plus the level of toxins present in our systems and how we treat ourselves. Together, these are responsible for our moods and general sense of wellness, as well as our ability to connect with our Divine source of love and wisdom.

Our hormones have a huge effect on our vibrancy. When hormones are out of balance, the entire body will be out of balance. Many factors affect hormones, ranging from food and water to too little or too much exercise, illness, thought patterns, emotions, the menstrual cycle, pregnancy, childbirth, menopause, gut flora, aging, the environment, and genetics — whew! As with illness, when our hormones are out of whack, we find it difficult to access Divine guidance.

Earlier I mentioned that food choices can profoundly affect our emotional states and, in turn, acts on our hormones and digestion, which (in a kind of loop) then influence our thoughts and feelings about food and thus what we consume. We can become caught up in a vicious cycle, causing us to eventually spiral down into the decrepit state that defines the later years of so many, as witnessed by the societal nightmare we refer to as nursing homes.

Perhaps you find yourself stuck in a Catch-22, whereby you eat poorly, which lowers your vibrancy, thereby disconnecting you from your intuition and hence an awareness of the importance of choosing foods that are beneficial for you. As a result of opting for things that have a negative impact on you, you feel emotionally depleted, which robs you of your motivation to love yourself, compounding the self-rejection and loneliness that sparked eating poorly in the first place.

The more we probe the functioning of the body, the more evident it becomes that what we take into ourselves — in the form of food and drink or through the body's interaction with the external environment — affects everything from the level of inflammation in our systems to how well our prefrontal cortex and amygdala function, regulating our energy, strength, stability of emotions, clarity of mind, ability to resist illness, and ability to connect with Divine guidance.

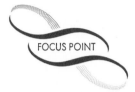

FOCUS POINT

The more we probe the functioning of the body, the more evident it becomes that what we take in affects everything in our system.

On a personal level, it comes down to whether you want to improve or degrade the quality of your life. Do you appreciate expanded perception and intuition, or are you going to allow excessive inflammation, insulin resistance, imbalance in the hypothalamic–pituitary-adrenal axis, metabolic issues, disrupted hormonal states, and impaired neurotransmitters — all of which are the result of nutrient depletion and the buildup of toxic waste — to leave you with decreased cognition, a disturbed emotional state, and a generally lowered level of consciousness?

A diet of quality foods augmented with other recognized promoters of health — such as adequate exercise and sleep and learning to manage stress in healthy ways (which I will teach you to do in the next section) — is a prime entry point for improving the quality of every aspect of our lives. Since the brain is one of the gateways connecting the body to the realm of the Divine, nourishing brain cells builds a solid foundation for deepening our spiritual connection.

While good nutrition supports a spiritual approach to life, it's conversely the case that a spiritual approach to life supports good nutrition. The more the mind, body, and soul are in harmony, the better we are at making wise food and lifestyle choices, as well as being able to carry through with them.

The goal is to live with an awareness of the unity of all life and to feel happy, healthy, and in harmony with all beings. More and more of us are making this a personal goal, and it needs to become a global goal. When we feel good, we transmit positive energy into the universe, influencing not just our well-beings but also the degree of joy experienced by everyone we meet. Imagine if this was how everyone lived. How different the world would be!

CHAPTER 8

DISCOVER THE RIGHT DIET FOR YOU

I've shown you that food — as well other substances, such as drugs and alcohol — has a huge effect on your digestive system and your state of well-being that depends on it. The industrialization and factory processing of food have led to not only illness but also emotional and spiritual disconnections. This lack of Divine connection is why so many of us feel alone, anxious, depressed, and empty inside. The toxicity caused by junk foods lowers our general state of health, reducing our vibrancy and thereby making it difficult to connect with the spiritual dimension of our nature from which springs the kind of meaningful guidance indigenous peoples experienced quite naturally.

How to Know What to Eat

It's when we get down to the nitty-gritty of what constitutes a healthy diet that matters aren't quite so simple. The fact is that it can be confusing to figure out how to eat for excellent health. I certainly was confused initially. It's not surprising, given that even the research is frequently contradictory.

"Eat more carbohydrates," one expert says, "especially more whole grains."

Another counters, "Don't eat grains because they are inflammatory," and advocates, "instead, eat more animal protein."

Other voices insist, "Don't eat meat. It causes cancer and heart disease. Become a vegetarian."

Someone else insists, "Of course you can eat meat, and you should, just as long as it's organic and pasture raised."

"No, don't eat animal products at all," a passionate group argues, "because the only healthy lifestyle is vegan."

Meanwhile others retort, "Vegan diet's aren't healthy. You'll end up malnourished."

There also are those who insist we should eat a specific kind of diet depending on our blood types, the climate we live in, and the time of year. Or we should eat in line with the eating habits of certain regions of the planet, as in the case of a Mediterranean diet or the diet advocated in *The China Study*.[1]

These widely touted viewpoints neglect the fact that we are all different, each with unique genetic predispositions, different metabolisms — yes, and even different blood types, as well as geographic variations because of the differences in the mineral content and so forth of the planet's soils. I'm not going to argue for a Paleo, vegetarian, vegan, raw food, or any other kind of diet. What I will suggest is that you start to notice whether you feel better with greater quantities of animal protein or greater quantities of vegetable protein or whether you feel better with greater quantities of animal fat or greater quantities of other healthy fats. Become conscious of what you are putting in your mouth and how it causes you to feel over a period of time. Allow your body to teach you and your intuition to guide you.

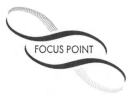
FOCUS POINT

Become conscious of what you are putting in your mouth and how it causes you to feel. Allow your body to teach you and your intuition to guide you.

---

1.   Colin Campbell (Dallas: BenBella Books, 2006).

If you find that eating vegan or vegetarian causes you to feel more alive, then study how to optimize these diets. If Paleo is your choice, be sure you know how and where what you eat was raised. Which-ever diet you select, allow the principle of eating as close to nature as possible to act as your guiding light. The intelligence of the universe knew what it was doing when it created our food, and our bodies are designed to utilize it. They are not designed to utilize the food-like manufactured products on the shelves of supermarkets.

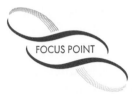

FOCUS POINT

Whichever diet you select, allow the principle of eating as close to nature as possible guide you. The intelligence of the universe knew what it was doing when it created our food, and our bodies are designed to utilize it.

Because of our different metabolisms, some of us might find we need animal protein to feel energized. If this is the case with you, be aware, as I previously stated, that studies have shown that eating grain-finished beef or lamb isn't good for anyone — that the fat of grain-finished animals is drastically altered in ways that can cause inflammation, which leads to impaired health. In contrast, the fat of organically raised, grass-fed, and grass-finished beef and lamb contains high quantities of omega-3, which isn't the case with grain-finished meat. In addition, livestock that graze on grass sprayed with pesticides have a high concentration of the pesticide in their fat, which leads to health problems. Also be sure to choose pastured organic poultry and eggs, as well as fish that's mercury-free and wild caught instead of farmed on manufactured feeds and dosed with antibiotics.

If you eat animal flesh, it's still important to make the centerpiece of your diet organic fruits and vegetables, which you can augment with soaked and sprouted organic nuts and seeds, sprouted organic beans, and sprouted organic whole grains — assuming that your body doesn't react with inflammation to any of these foods. Recent research indicates that, while meat contains a component called heme, which has been linked to cancer, green vegetables protect against malig-nancy. Dr. Sarah Ballantyne explains:

The link between red meat and cancer comes from diets that are simultaneously high in red meat (including high in processed meats) and low in green vegetables. The protection offered by green vegetables appears to be from chlorophyll ... which prevents the metabolism of a component of red meat (heme, which is much more concentrated in red meat than in other meats) into toxic products in the gut. Yet another reason to eat your greens![2]

Dairy is another controversial food. Many are sensitive to dairy and do best without it. However, I have found that some who can't tolerate pasteurized dairy find they do well on raw, pastured, organic dairy. Pasteurized dairy is inflammatory while raw, pastured, organic dairy is anti-inflammatory and healing for some people.[3]

I want to emphasize that when I made the commitment to eat healthily, I decided it was important to listen to my body. By tuning in to how different foods made me feel, I was able to discern the path to health that was appropriate for my body and my metabolism rather than buying into a particular food philosophy. To illustrate just how individual our bodies and metabolisms are, let me tell you about my client Marianne, who would fall asleep just fine but then awaken in a panic four to six hours later and find herself unable to go back to sleep.

Marianne understood that our thoughts create many of our feelings. She was vigilant when it came to keeping her thoughts constructive, having spent years practicing, so she couldn't understand why she was having such a hard time. Yet here she was, lying wide-awake in the middle of the night, night after night, ruminating about the various challenges in her life. After so much therapy, how could this be happening? That she had a deep spiritual connection and didn't, in any sense, feel alone in life made her dilemma all the more perplexing. She felt so out of control of her thoughts and feelings that she began to wonder whether she was going crazy. She had even tried

---

2. *The Paleo Approach* (Las Vegas: Victory Belt Publishing, 2014) p. 200.
3. Learn more about this at https://www.mindbodygreen.com/0-8646/the-dangers -of-dairy.html and https://www.realmilk.com/health/milk-cure/.

various forms of medication but found she wasn't responding well to any of the drugs.

"I just don't get what's happening," she bemoaned. "I take really great care of myself. I attend to my feelings, eat well, and exercise, and I have great friends and a wonderful relationship. My kids are doing well, and I love my work. Why am I having such a hard time?"

Because I had gone through the same experience, I suggested she ask her doctor to administer a glucose tolerance test. When a person's blood sugar drops too low, the adrenal glands take over and shoot epinephrine, also called adrenaline, into the system to send glucose to the brain, thus causing anxiety and even panic.

Sure enough, Marianne's functional medicine doctor confirmed the hypoglycemic diagnosis. Her doctor told her to go off all sugar and refined products such as white bread. She was also advised to eat often — at least six small meals per day, including lots of fruits and vegetables, healthy fats, and moderate amounts of protein. She explained to Marianne that while processed sugars and foods that turn into sugar in the body — like breads and pastas — will make her blood sugar issue worse, the natural sugar in fruit will help her blood sugar stabilize. While for many of us eating close to bedtime is inadvisable, the doctor advised her to be sure to eat a piece of fresh fruit just before going to sleep. Preferring to use alternative medicines whenever possible, the doctor further suggested she take a chromium supplement just before retiring for the night.

Within days of embracing this regimen, Marianne was sleeping through the night. On those occasions when she awakened, she was no longer anxious and was able to go back to sleep. Her depression also lifted. This worked well for a time. Then one night she again found herself not sleeping and, consequently, feeling anxious. When she shared this with me, I asked her, "What did you do differently during the day that preceded the night you couldn't sleep?"

"I joined a gym and did a hard workout," she explained. "I read that exercise is good for hypoglycemia." However, a little more research revealed that intense exercise greatly lowers blood sugar, which means she should not only eat some fruit before exercising but after as well. Also, the exercise might have dehydrated her, and the adrenals react the same way to dehydration as they do to low blood sugar. Marianne needed to be sure to drink enough water when she exercised. These simple adjustments ended her sleepless nights for good.

Tune in to Yourself to Determine the Effects of Foods

What types of foods energize you, and what types cause you to feel tired and depleted — not just in the short term, but also in the long run? Sugar and coffee can energize you for a while, but then the sugar will deplete you, as will the coffee if you don't do well on coffee. Some people have difficulty processing caffeine while others may actually benefit from it, especially when the coffee is organic. I can't drink more than a sip or two without feelings jittery and waking up with anxiety at night, whereas one of my clients was told by her functional medicine doctor to drink two cups a day to keep her blood pressure from being too low. This is a great example of how one size doesn't fit all. In fact, recent research shows that for some people, coffee is heart protective.[4]

Since most processed foods have little or no nutritional value, it's important to select foods that are nutrient dense — foods grown organically in healthy soil. Do you believe that eating healthy means choking down food you don't like? Nothing is further from the truth. Healthy food can be very delicious. I love the food I eat, and people who eat my food can't believe how delicious it is!

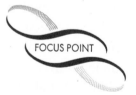

FOCUS POINT

Become aware of how foods affect you so that you can discover those that are right for you. Tune in to your body to learn which foods work to support your vibrancy and your Divine connection and which don't.

It can take some time to discover what you love and what is healthy for you, but you won't keep eating well if you don't love the food you eat. I suggest that you start a food diary. Write down everything you

---

4. See https://articles.mercola.com/sites/articles/archive/2017/09/11/coffee-beneficial -to-middle-aged-people.aspx.

eat, and keep track of how you feel right after, then hours later, and then even days later. Becoming aware of how food affects you is vital to discovering the foods that are right for you. If you learn to tune in to your body, your body will inform you about which foods work to support your vibrancy and your Divine connection and which don't:

Notice when your head feels foggy or fuzzy. Lack of mental clarity is often a symptom of a food reaction. If you have any candida in your system — which many people have because of too many antibiotics, a poor diet, overeating sugar or carbohydrates, or viruses — it can create fogginess. The candida fungus thrives on sugar, so anything that turns into sugar in the system (including nonfiber carbohydrates such as pasta and bread) feeds the candida.[5]

Pay attention when you suddenly feel a loss of energy. Certain foods that are not in alignment with your body can cause your body to work very hard to digest them, which causes a loss of energy. There are other foods that you might be allergic or sensitive to that can also rob you of energy.

Notice when you feel agitated, anxious, or panicked. Sometimes a certain food can trigger intense anxiety but not necessarily at the time you eat it. For example, if I drink caffeine or alcohol, I will wake up around 4:00AM with intense agitation and fear. The fear is not based on anything, but it's always easy to attach it to something that might be bothering me. The same thing occurs for me when I take an over-the-counter drug such as Tylenol PM. What relaxes many people has the opposite effect on me. It took me a while to figure this one out!

Notice when you feel depressed. Foods that you are allergic or sensitive to or that are not in harmony with your body can cause a feeling of depression. I've had clients who spent years trying to figure out the cause of their depression, and when they changed their diets, the depression went away.

Watch for symptoms such as congestion, itching, rashes, or dryness. These symptoms can be caused by the foods you are eating,

---

5.   Anthony William, *Medical Medium* (Carlsbad: Hay House, Inc., 2015), p. 119.
     Dr. Amy Myers, *The Autoimmune Solution* (San Francisco: HarperOne, 2015) pp. 82, 86, and 156.

or they could indicate a lack of something in your diet. For example, experiencing dryness might be due to a lack of healthy fats in the body, and having congestion could be due to pasteurized dairy products.

Notice your level of immunity. Do you catch colds or the flu often? Low immunity might indicate that your body is not getting what it needs to maintain optimal health.

Notice when it is difficult to feel Spirit within you. Certain foods could be lowering your vibrancy so much that you can't feel spiritual energy within you and around you. Food is, of course, just one aspect of vibrancy. Your vibrancy is also affected by your intention, thoughts, emotions, and behavior, which I address in part 3.

Notice how often you get hungry. Some people are rapid metabolizers and experience rapid transit, which means that they digest their food rapidly, and it's eliminated rapidly. These people need to eat more often to not be hungry or to not experience low blood sugar. Others are slow metabolizers, which means they don't have to eat as often. Notice whether you can go for long periods without feeling hungry or whether you feel hungry within two or three hours after eating.

I'm a rapid metabolizer, and I need to eat often. I will feel hungry two to three hours after eating, no matter how big my meal. Because of this, I bring plenty of my own food when I travel — also because I don't want to eat the junky airport or airplane food.

However, on a return plane trip in October 2016, we sat on the runway for twelve hours with an hour in the middle to eat. We changed from a defective plane to another plane, which also turned out to be defective, but it took forever for them to admit this to us. We were told over and over that we were leaving any minute, which we never did. The flight was canceled twelve hours from the scheduled departure time.

While I had enough of my food plus extra for my regular flight home, I didn't have enough for a whole day. There is only so much food you can take on a plane, so I was stuck eating at the airport. The airport food not only affected my vibrancy but also my skin and my sleep. It took me days to recover. Granted, I have a very sensitive body, but I know that everyone is being negatively affected to one degree or another, even if they are not aware of it.

What You Are Not Noticing

Many people are not motivated to eat well because they are not sensitive to or aware of the profound effects the food they eat has on them. They don't notice that their energy is a little lower or that they might not be as clearheaded. More importantly, they don't notice what junk food and devitalized foods are doing to their organs, immune system, and vibrancy. Then suddenly, one day — generally in their fifties, sixties, or seventies (and lately even in their twenties or thirties) — they notice it big time. This is when they might start to have health problems, such as heart disease, diabetes, cancer, or autoimmune diseases.

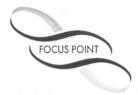

FOCUS POINT

Many people are in the habit of completely ignoring their feelings until they get sick. They don't notice that their moods, sleep patterns, stamina, pain levels, or connection with their higher selves are effected by the foods they eat.

While these health issues sometimes seem to come on suddenly, they have actually been developing during all their years of poor nutrition. They didn't notice because they didn't pay attention to how they felt physically, emotionally, and spiritually when they ate junk foods.

Many people are in the habit of completely ignoring their feelings. They don't notice that their moods, ability to sleep, stamina, pain levels, or ability to connect with their higher selves are affected by the food they eat. Often they just take a pill to relieve anxiety, depression, pain, or sleeplessness. Sometimes they drink more coffee to give them the energy to get through the day. In fact, they might use food to *avoid* their feelings rather than attend to them. Comfort food certainly works to make us feel better for the moment while covertly doing its damage in the body.

Here's an example of how unhealthy foods work on the body: Many of you know what happens to a frog when you put it in boiling water. It jumps out. But if you put it in cold water and then slowly heat it to boiling, the frog stays in the pot and dies. It is lulled into complacency by the slow rise in temperature. The same thing happens to many people regarding the foods they eat. They don't notice that damage is being done until they suddenly get sick.

Be Present in Your Body

It's a challenge for many people to be present in their bodies rather than focused in their minds. There is a good reason for this: Until you learn how to manage your emotions, it might be too scary to be present in your body with your feelings. However, until you are willing to be present in your body and notice the effects that food has on you, you might not be motivated to eat well.

When you truly desire a high level of health and a profound connection with your Divine guidance, then you will likely be motivated to eat well and enjoy a greater level of health and well-being instead of spending your later years dealing with illness and the feelings of aloneness and emptiness that are the result of spiritual disconnection.

If high energy, excellent health, and an inner spiritual connection are important to you, it's never too late to start noticing how you feel when you eat junk food as opposed to how you feel when you eat clean, fresh, organic foods. Notice how you feel when you take the time to make your meals from fresh ingredients as opposed to buying prepared packaged foods.

If you think you can't afford healthy food, think about how much money you will be saving on doctor bills and medications. See where you can cut back spending in other areas of your life. After all, what is more important in life than health and the fullness, love, and joy that come from Divine connection?

Test Your Food for Harmony

In *Power vs. Force*, David R. Hawkins, MD, PhD, tested levels of consciousness using kinesiology, also known as muscle testing. You can learn to use this technique to test which foods are harmonic with your body and support your health and which are dissonant and harmful to you.

It turns out that the muscles of the body respond to questions we ask or statements we make. For example, when I put my middle finger on my index finger (see figure 8.1) and push, the muscle of my index finger will stay strong or go weak, depending on what is true for me and what isn't. So when I say, "My name is Margaret," my finger stays strong, and when I say, "My name is Dan," my finger goes weak. This is just one way of muscle testing you can try. Many health practitioners test other muscles to discover what's going on in the body or what supplements you might need.[6]

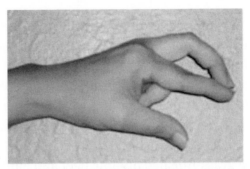

Finger positioning for muscle testing

You can use this technique to test foods and supplements. The way to do this is to hold a food in one hand while smelling it and putting it near your head, then your chest, and then your stomach while pushing on your index finger with your middle finger. If your index finger stays strong, then the food is likely fine for you, but if it goes weak, then it's not healthy for you. While this technique isn't always accurate (especially when you do it for yourself because your mind can get in your way), with practice, you can become quite good at it. I've used this many times when suspecting that something I was eating might not be right for me or when I wanted to try a new supplement.

This will not work when the food is in plastic. You need to either hold the food itself or hold it within glass. Plastic interferes with testing.

You can also use this to test the vibrancy of a food, but remember that we are all different. A high vibrancy, nutrient-dense food that might be great for someone else might not be in harmony with your

6.   To learn more about muscle testing, visit http://www.healing-with-eft.com/self -muscle-testing.html.

particular body and therefore isn't good for your health. Nevertheless, it's helpful to know in general which foods have a high vibrancy and which don't. Below is a list I have come up with regarding high and low frequency foods, but this is just my list. I encourage you to come up with your own.

My List of High-Vibrancy, Nutrient-Dense Foods (in Descending Order)

- fresh, local organic fruits and vegetables, especially dark leafy greens, grown on mineral-rich soil, and some dried fruits
- fermented organic vegetables and fruits
- healthy oils and fats — coconut, avocado, and olive oils; pastured organic ghee and butter; organic olives; organic avocados; pastured organic eggs; and the fat of pastured organic animals and wild-caught, oily, healthy fish
- grass-fed and grass-finished organic beef and lamb in moderation
- raw, organic dairy products, particularly fermented dairy, in moderation
- raw, soaked, sprouted, and low-heat organic dried nuts and seeds
- organic cacao
- sprouted organic grains: ancient forms of wheat, rice, quinoa, oats, rye, or barley in moderation (I am not sensitive to gluten)
- soaked organic legumes in moderation
- local organic honey and maple syrup in moderation

Local organic honey is excellent for healing allergies. Each time I've moved, I've been allergic to the new plants in the environment, but within weeks of eating 1 teaspoonful of local organic honey from bees within 25 miles of my house, the allergies are gone. Honey works homeopathically: There are very small amounts of all the plants in the area that the bees have been to for nectar, desensitizing the body to the allergens in your local environment.

My List of Low-Vibration, Low-Nutrient Foods

- sugar and high fructose corn syrup (HFCS)
- durum wheat
- factory-farmed meats and poultry

- pasteurized dairy
- factory-farmed fruits and vegetables grown on devitalized soil and sprayed with pesticides
- all foods grown from seeds that have been treated with genetically modified organisms (GMO)
- processed packaged foods and beverages, including sodas (even if organic) and gluten-free products
- all foods made with unhealthy oils — canola, corn, soybean, "vegetable," cottonseed, safflower, sunflower, and peanut

You can also ask your Divine guidance questions about which foods are right for you and which aren't. In the next section, you will learn more about how to connect with your Divine guidance with the second secret to Divine connection, but for now, just start with a deep desire to learn about what is for your highest good.

If you are suffering from a chronic illness, I strongly recommend that you read *The Autoimmune Solution* by Amy Myers, MD, and *The Wahls Protocol* by Terry Wahls, MD. While drugs are for symptoms, foods heal, and these writers will help you to understand what foods heal best. If you have or have had cancer, I recommend *The Gerson Therapy* by Dr. Charlotte Gerson.

CHAPTER 9

RECOVER YOUR WHOLENESS, AND RESTORE YOUR WELL-BEING

Since eating healthily is something so many of us fail at, it's worth asking what food means to us. Do we see it as a means of nourishing our bodies and thereby supporting us in excellent health, or do we regard it primarily as a means of satisfying our various cravings? Is eating an experience we enjoy, even relish, but don't abuse with wrong or excessive foods? Or is eating a way to mask feeling uncomfortable, lonely, anxious, or emotionally distressed in some other way? In other words, do we eat to suppress sensations and emotions we don't like, utilizing food and beverages to "numb out" in the way a pacifier or blanket comforts an infant?

In my early twenties, I lived with my aunt, who always had a cake or two in her freezer. I used to sneak frozen cake, little pieces at a time, hoping she wouldn't notice. I just had to get my sugar fix. Then I started to read about nutrition and realized how toxic sugar is for the body. Exercising all the willpower I could muster, I was determined to clean up my act. I would stop eating sugar, period.

After several attempts, I actually managed to go off it completely for two years. The problem was that the craving didn't go away. After a few months of abstention, it lessened somewhat. Thinking I was cured, I made the mistake of taking just one bite of a sugary treat, and my craving was revived full-blown. I should add that along with my sugar addiction, I struggled on and off with my weight.

Are you addicted to self-medicating with sugar? Or perhaps your addiction is to baked goods, junky fast food, too much food, alcohol, smoking, over-the-counter pharmaceuticals, or even illegal drugs. If this is the case, do you find you are unable to stop using these substances? It can be extremely difficult to kick any kind of addiction when the addiction masks painful feelings that you've never learned to lovingly manage.

Alcohol, tobacco, pills, and illegal substances were never my issue, but I've worked with countless clients who were addicted to such substances. For me the problem was simply sugar. Like bees to nectar, I was drawn to its sweetness.

When I was growing up, my grandmother lived with us. One of the things I remember vividly about her is that she always had a piece of hard candy in her mouth. Today I understand that this is how she soothed herself. Constantly sucking on a piece of candy was a source of comfort, akin to sucking on a pacifier. Based on what health researchers are currently disclosing concerning the effects of sugar on the body, I have no doubt that ingesting so much candy contributed to her dying of pancreatic cancer when she was seventy-six years old. I'm also confident that growing up around someone who sucked on sugar all day fueled my sugar addiction.

When I was intensely sugar addicted, I craved it all the time. The more I ate, the more I craved it. It didn't seem to matter that it made me feel terrible. I'd experience the high; then after a while, I'd crash and find myself spaced out. I loathed feeling this way, but that didn't deter me because I craved my sugar more than I cared about how I felt.

In time I discovered that sugar was my fix for anxiety, which I often felt. This anxiety was often accompanied by a feeling of aloneness, which in turn made me more anxious — sometimes to the point that my anxiety all but consumed me. In those days, I didn't understand that these feelings of aloneness and anxiety were the result of having abandoned myself in various ways, resulting in being disconnected from my core soul self and my Divine guidance. Today I recognize that this was true not only of me but also of a great many of us.

As a child, my spontaneous, authentic self was viewed by grown-ups as far too exuberant, which meant that I frequently experienced adults squelching my natural enthusiasm for life. This resulted in my feeling rejected by those who were most significant to me. At times I felt abandoned by them, as if I perhaps should never have intruded on their worlds. It was this crushing of my core self that left me not only feeling alone but also anxious about my very existence and my place in the scheme of things.

Feeling so doubtful about my validity led to years of having unloving thoughts about myself. Over the course of a couple of decades, I said some awful things about me to myself. I often acted in ways that were anything but kind to myself, which frequently provoked others to behave in an equally unloving manner toward me. In many ways, these were very painful years.

While most of us have experienced the alone or empty feeling I'm referring to, and we certainly know what it is to be anxious, few of us realize that, as adults, the self-abandonment causing these feelings is often the root of our issues with eating and drinking unhealthily. What I soon discovered is that all unloving behavior we have toward ourselves — together with the aloneness, emptiness, anxiety, and depression we endure when we don't feel good about ourselves — dissipates when we at last discover and connect with our rejected and abandoned core selves and our Divine guidance, as do the issues we have with addiction to food and drink, along with other substances and addictive behaviors.

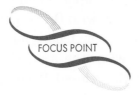

FOCUS POINT

Few of us realize that, as adults, the self-abandonment that causes our feelings of emptiness and anxiety is often the root of our issues with eating and drinking unhealthily.

Food addiction can be difficult to deal with because we can't just stop eating. One client, Hannah, for example, was distressed that with all the inner work she had done, she still found herself binge eating.

"There are times when I just can't quit munching," she confided.

"I feel awful afterward, but at the time, I just want another cookie and another until they're all gone. Or I'll intend to take a few bites of ice cream out of the carton and find myself unable to stop until the carton is empty. I don't get why I'm still doing this. It seems worse since I married Bernard even though I really love him. I can't figure this out."

I asked Hannah to tune in to the addicted part of herself and allow that part to speak about why she needed to fill up with food.

After several moments she responded, "Sometimes I feel so empty and alone inside. I just can't stand it. The food makes me feel so much better. I don't feel so alone when I'm eating and filled up. But I don't get why I feel this way. I'm not alone; I have Bernard, and he loves me. Why do I feel alone inside when I'm not alone outside?"

We'll return to Hannah's story and how she moved on from binge eating toward the end of the book. For now, I simply want to point out that most people think the empty feeling is caused by something outside them, such as not having a partner, feeling rejected by someone, being unhappy in their jobs, or not having enough money. But this is never what causes inner emptiness and the feeling of aloneness we experience.

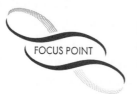

FOCUS POINT

Most people think the empty feeling is caused by something outside them, but this is never what causes inner emptiness and feeling alone.

I need to be clear about my use of terminology, since people use the terms "alone," "aloneness," and "lonely" differently. An acute feeling of inner aloneness or emptiness is the result of self-abandonment. We are missing our true selves and our connection with Divine guidance. This is different from simply being alone or from feeling lonely. We might feel lonely when we want to connect with others and there is no one around or when the person we are with is closed. We might also feel lonely when we are closed, because we can't connect when our hearts are closed.

We are social creatures who value contact with others. Some of us, those of us who are more extroverted, thrive when we have lots of people in our lives, whereas those of us who are more introverted like to spend a great deal of our time alone. These are personal preferences based on who we are in our soul essence, neither better than the other. We don't feel alone and empty inside when we are connected with our soul essence and with our Divine guidance. It's when we abandon ourselves that we can feel alone and empty inside, even when we are with others; however, choosing to be alone at times can be perfectly enjoyable.

Believe You Are Worth Loving Enough to Eat Well

We take good care of what we value. When we indulge in sugar and processed foods, we abandon ourselves by rejecting a crucial aspect of ourselves — a healthy body for our souls to express through. When we physically abandon ourselves by putting unhealthy food into our bodies, the message we send to ourselves is that we aren't worth taking loving care of. The question is why would anyone feel this way about themselves?

All the ways we abandon ourselves, including eating those foods that harm us, stem from feeling unseen, devalued, and unloved as we were growing up, creating the big empty hole inside us that I've been referring to — the hole where our true selves are meant to be. Unfortunately, it was suppressed as a result of the things that happened (or failed to happen) in childhood. The ways we learned to abandon ourselves also stem from the role modeling we experienced from our parents or other caregivers in how they treated themselves. Do you tend to treat yourself the way you were treated or the way your role models treated themselves?

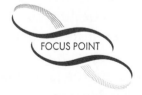

FOCUS POINT

We take good care of what we value. When we physically abandon ourselves by putting unhealthy food into our bodies, the message we send to ourselves is that we aren't worth taking loving care of.

When we feel alone or empty inside, it's because we are abandoning ourselves and then experiencing the void where our true selves are meant to be continuously blossoming. Without a loving connection with our true selves, we don't feel complete. This inner emptiness leaves us longing for something or someone to fill the hole.

Wanting to share our lives with others is healthy. At the same time, it can (in part) be a manifestation of an insatiable neediness stemming from feeling empty or alone inside because our real selves are unknown to us and because we are abandoning ourselves rather than loving ourselves. What fills that emptiness is love — our love for ourselves. But when we don't know our real selves, it's hard to want to love ourselves.

If we find we are desperate for junk food or another addiction or for someone to fill up our emptiness (which is a far more acute sensation than simply enjoying being close to another), it may be that we are anxious to escape feeling the void inside us where our true selves ought to be feeling loved by us. The presence of someone who can be counted on to fill the emptiness renders our neediness somewhat tolerable, but it's a far cry from sharing love.

As we move into the years when we entertain committing to a partner, the emptiness caused by the absence of knowing and loving our authentic selves and our connection with the Divine can also be what's behind the longing for a partner. It's worth exploring whether such a desire is healthy (it can indeed be) or a desperate need for someone to make us feel worthy and to fill the emptiness and aloneness we feel.

What's going on in a situation where attachment to another is based on a deep neediness is that the other provides us with the love and attention that we haven't learned to give ourselves. The person becomes a substitute for the love we are not giving to our soul essence — our authentic selves. We need to relate to others and share love with them, but the less we connect with ourselves, the harder time we have connecting with others in a healthy manner. We cannot share love when we abandon ourselves. Instead, we keep trying to get the love we need to feel safe and worthy within.

Because our authentic selves might have been lost to us since childhood, so overwhelming is the sense of abandonment at times that we might even feel alone when we're with someone to whom we feel close. We might be in the same room, even the same bed, and still feel lonely because we can't connect with the person when we are disconnected from ourselves.

What do we do in situations when another isn't available to alleviate our distress or perhaps is available and we still feel distressed?

Many of us eat or drink — and usually not healthy food and beverages. In an attempt to avoid the pain of our self-abandonment and to plug the hollow feeling inside us, we turn to junk. If we don't head for fast food, maybe we sit on the couch and eat a bag of chips, devour a whole package of cookies, or indulge in an ice cream fest. We also chug soft drinks or attempt to douse our inner longings with liquor or drugs.

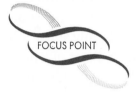

FOCUS POINT

We need to relate to others and share love with them, but the less we connect with ourselves, the harder time we have connecting with others in a healthy manner.

The result, at least in the Western world, is that we are witnessing a generation in which large numbers of us are overweight, with no small percentage of us classified as outright obese — a condition that not many years ago was a rarity. Alcoholism has also become a huge problem not only for adults but also our youth. Simultaneously we are seeing more people with degenerative diseases, particularly cancer, diabetes, and autoimmune diseases. The reason for this goes beyond the fact that many are addicted to sugar, as I was, as well as to junk foods. The sad fact is that despite the abundance available to us as in no other era, even foods normally considered healthy — including fruits and vegetables — fail to provide us with the nutrition they supplied to people just a generation or two ago, grown as they are on artificial fertilizers in denatured soils and sprayed with toxic pesticides. To compound the situation, more of us lead sedentary lives, working in office jobs in which sitting is the main way our day is spent and sunlight hardly ever touches our skin.

Food is often the primary go-to form of self-medicating for many, not just because it's readily available, but also because much of it has been laced with addictive substances. Sugar obviously is the most prevalent, though far from the only harmful and addictive additive.

Eating and drinking are ways we continue to abandon ourselves, recapitulating the abandonment we endured in childhood. We eat and drink in such a manner as to desert ourselves, using food and beverages to mask the inner aloneness, emptiness, anxiety, and lack of self-love that torment us. Doing this, we abandon our health and well-being — and thus betray our very souls.

Reawaken Your Core Essence

Now, are you ready for some truly good news? Our core selves are the homes to our unique gifts and talents, passionate purposes, natural wisdom and intuition, curiosity, sense of wonder, playfulness, spontaneity, and our abilities to love and connect with others. This is the unwounded aspect of our souls. There is a part of the soul that can never be harmed. It has never been touched by any abuse we suffered. Instead, this core aspect of us — this essence of our being — became hidden away and waits to be retrieved through the process of awakening.

It's because of this unbroken part we each have that healing past hurts can occur, no matter how severe. The entirety of our pasts becomes integrated with our beings, orchestrated by our souls and Divine guidance so that in the end, we become an integrated whole. This is the experience of wellness, well-being, and wholeness.

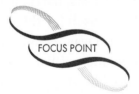

FOCUS POINT

A part of the soul can never be harmed and is untouched by any abuse you've experienced. That part of your soul waits for your awakening.

The key to robust health and well-being, which requires the ability to maintain an ongoing commitment to the kind of diet and lifestyle that's right for you — shown to you through your connection to the Divine — is to recover the whole of who you are. This entails reawakening what I variously refer to as our essence, our authentic selves, our true selves, our core selves, our awakened selves, or our essential beings. I'm speaking of the aspect of the soul we learned to disown when we were little.

Enjoying tiptop health requires us to engage in the process of reclaiming our core selves and learning to connect with our Divine guidance. The wellness, well-being, and wholeness that results become apparent as we increasingly retrieve, learn to deeply know, and come to value this feeling aspect of ourselves above all else. We at last recognize who we really are as children of the unconditional love that is God — or the Great Spirit, the Universe, or whichever concept works best for you.

To be made aware of the hollowed-out feeling you might experience until you awaken to the presence of your true being — your core — and let go of the various addictions covering up your pain can be challenging. The reason we're addicted to whatever causes us to feel temporarily satisfied — food (especially sugar, starches, and chemicalized junk), alcohol, tobacco, narcotics, and the like — is that these are substitutes for our true selves until the authentic version emerges, which finally fills us up and, in due course, overflows to everyone around us.

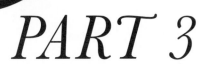

PART 3

INTENTION: THE SECOND SECRET TO DIVINE CONNECTION

Heal Your Diet of Junk Thoughts and
Unloving Actions, and Learn
to Love Yourself

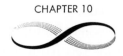

CHAPTER 10

TAKE RESPONSIBILITY FOR YOUR FEELINGS

I ate extremely well for years, but I still struggled with my Divine connection. It wasn't until I learned to consciously open to learning about loving myself that I could connect with my guidance at will, as well as refine my diet in a manner that was optimal for me. As long as I abandoned myself — not even knowing I was doing so — my vibrancy was too low to connect with my Divine guidance, even with my excellent diet.

When I sought out therapy to help me solve the difficulties I was having in my marriage, it was because I wanted to learn what I was doing to cause my husband to be angry with me and at times shut down. Like so many women, I believed that when he was unloving to me, it was my fault.

Though I was the equivalent of Mother Earth for not only my husband but also our three children and my parents, none of the different approaches therapists recommended changed either the situation or how unhappy I felt. I believed something was very, very wrong with me. I also believed there had to be something I could do about it, but that "something" eluded me. To get to the root of my problems, the therapists I saw focused not only on how I might improve things but they also took me deep into my childhood in an attempt to get to the reasons for my marital pain.

It wasn't just in my immediate family that I was having problems. Whenever anyone disconnected from me, sometimes completely rejecting me, I felt utterly baffled by why it was happening, and I became very upset by it. I remembered many things about my past during these years of therapy, but it did nothing to change things to help me understand my current unhappy experiences. The one thing that seemed clear to me was that what I was experiencing was somehow my fault, and if only I could change, then I would be loved.

Well, it turned out that it was my fault, but it was for a reason very different from what any of the therapists considered. Through all the forms of counseling during those many years, not one of the therapists suggested that other people were treating me the way I treated myself. Neither did anyone tell me that I wasn't responsible for my husband's behavior — that it wasn't my job to try to keep him happy. Only he could do this for himself. I had been making the mistake of taking responsibility for everyone's feelings but my own.

Growing up, I had unwittingly become a master of self-rejection; so many of us do! The fact that I needed to stop rejecting myself was just never discussed throughout my entire experience of psychoanalysis or the many other forms of therapy I tried.

My one constant companion in life up to this point was a sense of shame. The idea that feeling ashamed of myself and being self-critical were forms of rejecting myself didn't occur to me. In fact, realizing that abandoning myself was the real cause of my troubles came as a shock.

I was seven years into my marriage when a profound discovery changed my life: At any given moment, I was directed by only one of two intentions: (1) to learn about loving myself and others or (2) to protect myself against pain with some form of controlling behavior (such as turning to food and various other addictions to numb myself) and giving myself up to control others. When I learned to be aware of my intention and that I could choose to open to learning about loving myself, I finally understood the two secrets to attaining ongoing, at-will Divine connection. What a reversal this insight was of everything I had believed about myself!

I was convinced that by sacrificing myself to cater to others, I was being loving. Suddenly I saw that all my efforts to get others to love me were an exercise in control that was not only futile but also caused me a lot of pain.

The Power of Shame

I made the decision to notice my self-judgments. The key to this was to pay attention to when I became anxious, especially around people. I noticed that my anxiety was caused primarily by my self-judgments about not being good enough. It took me a year of consistently noticing how I put myself down before I was finally able to stop criticizing myself. Then in a surprise "aha!" moment, I became aware that shaming myself with self-judgments and trying to control other people's feelings about me and how they acted toward me were intricately linked.

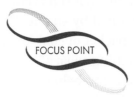

FOCUS POINT

The ego — the wounded part of us whose whole definition revolves around fear and control — is terrified of losing control.

I saw that shaming myself through self-criticism was a way to control myself to do the "right" things, say the "right" things, behave the "right" way, and look "right" so that I could have control over how others felt about me. I saw that my wounded ego was deeply addicted to controlling me as well as trying to control others.

The ego — the wounded part of us whose whole definition revolves around fear and control — is terrified of losing control. But even as it seeks to control, it is equally fearful of being controlled. Our ego-wounded selves deeply fear losing us through being controlled and losing others through rejection. At the same time, this wounded aspect of us is incapable of setting appropriate limits against engulfment or dealing with rejection in healthy ways.

My client Lauren quickly discovered the difference between control and setting meaningful limits. When she first came to see me, she was borderline diabetic and had been advised by her doctor to avoid candy, cookies, soft drinks, and other forms of sugar. She had tried everything, including Overeaters Anonymous, in her determination to give up her addiction to sugar, but nothing worked. The more she failed at diet plan after diet plan, the more ashamed she felt.

Seeing her deep sense of shame, I decided to take a different route from addressing her consumption of sugary foods directly. Instead, we worked on her self-judgments and her boundary issues. As she shared the details of her life with me, it became apparent that for years she had allowed everyone significant in her life to control her — her husband, her son, and her siblings. As I shared this insight with her and the truth of it dawned on her, she began to notice how often she judged herself and how much this led to being treated badly by others. As a result of starting to feel better about herself and of learning to have compassion for her feelings and forgiveness for her unloving behavior toward herself, she began to learn to set loving limits on losing herself through giving herself up to others.

Three months after she had started seeing me, Lauren arrived at one of our sessions all smiles, no longer consumed by shame. "It's a month today since I ate my last candy bar and packet of cookies," she announced proudly. "I haven't even craved anything sugary."

Lauren's craving for a sugar high had come from feeling inwardly abandoned whenever she let others, especially her husband, run over her. As long as she took care of herself by firmly (but with a kind tone) speaking up for herself and taking loving action for herself, she had no desire to further harm her health and end up a full-blown diabetic.

From my experiences and my years of working with my clients, I can promise you that if you let go of your need to control how others feel about you by selling yourself out in an attempt to please them — or by getting angry, blaming, and being judgmental in an effort to control them — and instead move into compassion (first for yourself and then for those around you), you'll let go of the false beliefs about your inadequacies and begin to feel empowered. You'll stop constantly apologizing for yourself because you feel ashamed. You'll also find that you begin to take care of your health by eating well.

To discover our beautiful soul essence and learn to love ourselves, we need to become aware of why and how we are not loving ourselves and why and how we are rejecting and abandoning ourselves. As I previously stated, we take good care of what we value, and we tend to avoid, reject, and abandon what we don't value. What happened that led to our lack of self-value — of not knowing the beauty and wonderfulness of our true soul selves?

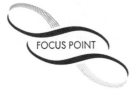

FOCUS POINT

To discover our beautiful soul essence and learn to love ourselves, we need to become aware of why and how we are not loving ourselves and why and how we are rejecting and abandoning ourselves.

As children, if we don't receive the love we need, we are incapable of recognizing that the issue is our parents' inability to love us, which includes helping us learn self-regulation regarding our feelings. We are too young to comprehend that their failure to do so has nothing to do with us. Instead, we conclude that it's somehow our fault, which can lead to a lifelong feeling that we're simply not good enough. Shame is the feeling that we can never do anything right because there's something fundamentally wrong with us. This is quite different from guilt.

The feeling of guilt involves doing something wrong or at least imagining we're doing something wrong. Whether we really are is another matter, since we can feel guilty for going against something someone laid on us as a great truth when in fact it's completely false.

Shame is a feeling that we are "wrong" at our core. It's feeling that it's not okay to be ourselves. At some point, we unconsciously decide that we are not being loved because we are inherently flawed, inadequate, defective, and consequently unimportant, undeserving, and unworthy of love.

This isn't something we articulate. We're much too young to draw such conscious conclusions. It's a sense of ourselves that we pick up from not feeling seen, understood, valued, and loved. Had we been capable of recognizing our parents' limitations to love us, we would have felt crushingly helpless, and we might have even given up on life. Instead of giving up, most of us choose to try to control the situation in an attempt to get someone to love us. But what control do we have at such a young age?

Shaming ourselves is one thing that gives us a sense of control.

We tell ourselves that our parents' attitude and behavior toward us are our fault because of our defectiveness. If their behavior is our fault, then, we conclude, we can change ourselves to be what they want us to be to get their approval. This results in hiding who we really are — our beautiful soul selves — and devoting our energy to figuring out how to be the kind of person that will get us the love we crave while simultaneously avoiding the heartbreak and loneliness of their inability to love us adequately, since we are incapable of handling it at this age.

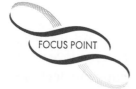

FOCUS POINT

Shaming ourselves is one thing that gives us a sense of control.

The Importance of Self-Worth

If we believe we are inherently defective, what choice do we have but to hide our real selves as we struggle to behave in ways we imagine will make us acceptable and therefore lovable? As we lose touch with ourselves, we adopt an image of the person we think we're supposed to be in order to be lovable. We call this self-image the ego, which I've been referring to throughout this book primarily as in connection with our wounded condition.

The ego — the wounded self — is a created version of us that can be quite far from the essential self. We find that we are stuck defining ourselves through such things as our looks, intelligence, popularity, or performance, which are naturally accompanied by the anxiety that comes from being so vulnerable to the disapproval of those who are important to us. Because our wounded selves feel worthy only when receiving validation from others, our very existence can unwittingly come to revolve around trying to look the "right" way, say the "right" thing, and do the "right" thing. Our whole existence is geared to getting others to like us, approve of us, and love us.

In some cases the ego generates a powerful drive that takes people to the peak of what the world considers success. But it doesn't come with the natural, easy flow of our authentic selves. Frequently it's about proving our worth to others and often to ourselves. Is it any wonder we experience so much anxiety? How can we possibly feel safe when our whole sense of worth hinges on others' approval?

I hear some form of "I'm not good enough" from most of my clients. It might show up a bit differently in each person, but the underlying belief is the same:

"I have no value."

"I'm not good enough, and I will never be good enough."

"I'm stupid."

"I'm a loser."

"I'm flawed; there is really something fundamentally wrong with me."

"I don't like myself."

"If he or she doesn't like me, there must be something wrong with me."

"If they really knew me, they wouldn't like me."

"I don't deserve to be loved."

"I'm not important."

"I am not lovable."

"I am unworthy and undeserving of love."

"It is my fault that he or she doesn't like me."

"If someone rejects me, it must be my fault."

"I am inadequate."

"I'll never get this right. I'll never be okay."

"I am a failure. I will never amount to anything."

"I am ugly. I am too tall, too short, too fat, too thin, too dark, too light," and so on.

"I am selfish when I take care of myself."

"I am alone, and I will always be alone. I'm one of those people meant to be alone."

"No one will ever love me."

When children are ridiculed, taunted, bullied, or physically or sexually abused by parents, teachers, siblings, and other children, they absorb a sense of shame that compounds their feelings of inadequacy. Instead of realizing the abusers are wrong about them, they grow up believing they are worthless. For example, a client named

Lindsay shared that when she was a girl, her father constantly put her down, assaulted her with a belt, and touched her inappropriately while her mother did nothing to protect her from the abuse. The family sat around the dinner table as if nothing of the kind was going on, all the while criticizing Lindsay for her sullenness.

If you are told over and over that you're ugly, that you shouldn't have been born, and that you are a bother and a burden, how can you possibly escape feeling you have no value? Especially when school bullies pick up on your low self-worth and torment you mercilessly, as happened to Lindsay, you're bound to feel worthless. If at the same time you are being abused or molested, the shame you experience is compounded many times over.

Self-Inflicted Shame

As bad as shame feels, many prefer to be in control of inflicting shame on themselves than feeling painful experiences, which happen in varying degrees in everyone's life, such as loneliness, heartbreak, grief, sadness, sorrow, helplessness concerning others, and feeling crushed or shattered. Just as anger is often a cover-up for these feelings, so is shame. Shame is a feeling we inflict on ourselves from our false beliefs, whereas the painful experiences I listed are a natural part of life.

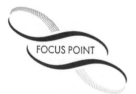

As bad as shame feels, many prefer to inflict it on themselves than feel painful experiences, which happen in varying degrees in every life.

We feel grief over losing someone we love and lonely when we want to connect or play with someone and there's no one available. We feel heartbroken, crushed, or shattered when someone important to us is being mean to us and especially if we lose someone we love.

On one hand, others shame us, and on the other, we frequently shame ourselves. Because we weren't shown how to handle painful feelings when we were children, many of us would prefer to feel an awful feeling that *we are causing* rather than experience life in its raw reality. What we don't realize is that shaming ourselves is also something we might be addicted to. Repeatedly rejecting ourselves by avoiding or stuffing away our feelings of loneliness and helplessness concerning others easily leads to addictive behavior. Abandoning ourselves for our various addictions eventually results in despair.

Let's go back to Lindsay's story for a moment. We met her a short while ago. As happened in my life, there came a point when she was tired of feeling bad about herself. To change how she felt, she needed to fully acknowledge what had happened in her childhood. I can't tell you how often the people I work with trivialize and diminish what happened to them as children. "Oh, it wasn't that bad," they'd tell me. "I'm sure many had it worse than I did." Trivializing or diminishing what happened is akin to a child coming to you to report abuse and you responding, "I don't believe you" or "It's no big deal; get over it."

As I helped Lindsay acknowledge how lonely, helpless, heartbroken, crushed, and shattered she felt as a child, she cried for the first time in years. Rather than continuing to blame and judge herself, she began to feel compassion and forgiveness toward herself for having been so judgmental. As she did so, she found herself spontaneously opening up to her core self and, consequently, for the first time in her life, treating herself as the sweet, kind, caring person she is by nature.

What I'm about to say might be a little difficult to grasp at first: If you find it difficult to move beyond shame and the self-judgments that cause it, it's because you are addicted to the appearance of control it gives you. You've bought into the illusion that you can control others' feelings and behaviors, and by so doing, you can mitigate the potential distress of rejection. Shaming yourself allows you to continue the illusion that others' unloving behavior toward you is your fault, and if only you change, you can have control over being loved and accepted. Shame actually disappears when you fully accept your helplessness concerning others' feelings and behavior. Take a moment to ponder this.

I don't wish to imply that beginning to feel your real feelings instead of masking them with dysfunctional behavior isn't uncomfortable at first. I certainly didn't find it comfortable, and neither have many of my clients, including Lindsay. So let me briefly take you through what's involved by relating the experience of another of my clients, Marilee.

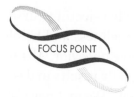

FOCUS POINT If you find it difficult to move beyond shame and self-judgments, it's because you are addicted to the appearance of control they give you.

When Marilee was seven, her aunt (her mother's sister) died in a car accident. Never having learned to manage her big painful feelings, Marilee's mother couldn't handle her grief. Instead, she shut down and turned to alcohol to numb herself. In shutting down to her pain, she also shut down to Marilee and Marilee's younger brother.

Marilee initially came to me for help because of her own excessive drinking. She knew she was harming herself, yet her willpower faltered again and again whenever she tried to reduce her imbibing. As she started to work with me, I observed that she was like a talking head with no connection to her body. Most of the time it was as if she were unaware she even had a body.

When we lose touch with our essence, it doesn't give up on us. Rather, it seeks ways to come alive. It's no surprise, then, that Marilee was addicted to seeking out relationships in which she used sex in an attempt to connect. During sex, she felt momentarily alive and in her body, connected with her partner, but inevitably that feeling was short-lived. Because she was emotionally detached, every relationship she attempted rapidly became boring. There was no way to maintain the connection when she lived from her head rather than from her heart and soul.

We can't shut down to our pain without also shutting down to our wonderful core feelings such as love, compassion, peace, and joy. Marilee learned that just having an orgasm is very different from the rapture of sexual bliss in a relationship infused with heartfelt connection.

Like Marilee, I learned to stay focused in my head as a means of disconnecting from my pain. I was aware of my anxiety, anger, guilt, shame, and (at times) depression, but I had no idea that I was causing these feelings as a result of my self-judgment and self-rejection.

Define Your Core Self

What will motivate you to stop rejecting yourself by judging and shaming yourself? If you are a junk food junkie or you frequently fail to eat well, can you see how such a diminished existence is the result of the shame you feel? If you are one of those who are unconcerned about nutrition, what shaming in your past lies behind this lack of concern for your well-being?

When you treat yourself in ways that will likely lead to a future painful health issue, you are practicing self-rejection. Is your health important to you? If not, the shame that has you in its grip will cause you to go right on physically and emotionally abandoning yourself. When you are no longer driven by shame, you'll be empowered to make healthy choices, which will affect every aspect of your well-being and the quality of your entire life. We heal from shame when we do the following:

- We accept that we aren't the cause of others' feelings unless we are being unloving to them, and we don't cause their unloving behavior toward themselves or toward us. We can't control them by changing ourselves.
- We learn to lovingly manage our existential painful feelings of loneliness, heartbreak, grief, and helplessness concerning others so that we no longer need to avoid them by covering them up with our self-judgments, which is what causes our shame.
- We learn to define our intrinsic worth.

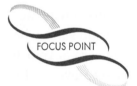

FOCUS POINT

When you are no longer driven by shame, you'll be empowered to make healthy choices, which will affect every aspect of your well-being and the quality of your entire life.

When we embrace the intention to learn, one of the things we need to learn about is who we really are. However, we can't know this through the mind's eyes — the eyes of the wounded self who is filled with false beliefs. We can know who we truly are only through the eyes of truth — the eyes of Divine guidance. When we look at ourselves through the eyes of truth, we can move beyond defining our worth externally and learn to see who we are internally. Defining yourself internally means opening to learning about your core self.

Try the following to connect with Divine guidance:

- At a time when you feel peaceful and relaxed, take some deep breaths.

- Become centered in your heart.
- Picture your Divine guidance. Imagine that your guidance is with you. It is surrounding you and within you.
- Ask your guidance to show you what your guidance sees and loves about you — your true self.
- Imagine that you can see your soul essence, your beautiful inner child, through the eyes of your Divine guidance — the eyes of love.
- Look into your inner child's eyes and see who you really are. See your light, goodness, innocence, vulnerability, aliveness, and lovingness. See how precious your inner child is, how inherently lovable. See that your inner child is worthy of being loved and cared for by you. See that this child just wants to be loved and be loving.
- Try to imagine who you were before your wounded self took over — who you were as a child. Were you loving, caring, fun, alive, creative, sensitive, and passionate?
- If you could have you as your child, what would you value in that child? Would the child be worthy in your eyes only if he or she performed right or looked right, or would you see inside to who this child really is?

Defining your intrinsic worth is one of the most loving actions you can take for yourself. It's when you deeply love and value who you truly are that you will be motivated to take loving care of your body, the house of your beautiful soul. The more you see, love, and value yourself, the more your addictions will naturally fall away.

Part of defining your essence is noticing, throughout the day, what you do that is loving, kind, creative, and funny. Notice when you are curious, and appreciate that. Start to notice the qualities in yourself that you appreciate in others.

Defining your worth is an ongoing process, not a one-time experience. The more you tune in to your feelings — your inner guidance — and to your higher guidance, the more you will come to see and appreciate your true, intrinsic self.

CHAPTER 11

THE WAYS YOU ABANDON YOURSELF

If you feel alone, empty, anxious, depressed, hurt, angry, jealous, sad, fearful, guilty, or shame, it's likely that you are rejecting and abandoning yourself in numerous ways. If you are acting out with substance or process addictions or experiencing relationship or parenting problems, it's likely you are abandoning yourself.

These issues are frequent results of self-abandonment. The Encarta World English Dictionary defines "abandon" as follows: *to leave somebody or something behind for others to look after, especially somebody or something meant to be a personal responsibility.*

As an adult capable of taking care of yourself, you cannot be abandoned by another person, since they are not responsible for you. We can abandon a child, an ill person, or an old person — someone who cannot care for themselves and whom we have agreed to care for. But if you are a physically healthy and sane adult, you can be left, but others cannot abandon you. Only *you* can abandon you.

Do you reject yourself, making others responsible for you and then feel abandoned when they leave you or don't take responsibility for you? As adults, our well-being is our personal responsibility. Others can love us, support us, and help us to heal, but as long as we reject ourselves, their love will not heal the shame that comes from rejecting and abandoning ourselves. There are many ways we have learned to abandon ourselves emotionally, physically, financially, organizationally, spiritually, or relationally:

- staying focused in your mind and ignoring your feelings rather than being present in your body
- judging, criticizing, and shaming yourself
- turning to various addictions as a way of numbing yourself and avoiding responsibility for learning from and lovingly managing your feelings
- making others responsible for your feelings of worth and safety
- eating badly
- not exercising
- not sleeping well
- procrastinating
- overspending
- underspending, even when money is available
- being consistently late, always disorganized, or living in clutter
- not participating in a spiritual practice
- giving yourself up to others
- not speaking up for yourself
- using anger, blame, judgment, or violence to try to control others

This is certainly not a complete list. Anything we do that results in feeling depressed, anxious, or shamed could be a form of self-abandonment.

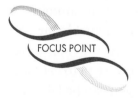

FOCUS POINT

As adults, our well-being is our personal responsibility. Other can love us, support us, and help us to heal, but as long as we reject ourselves, their love will not heal our shame that comes from rejecting and abandoning ourselves.

Emotional Self-Abandonment

What are the ways you might be emotionally rejecting and abandoning yourself? I've identified four major ways:

- self-judgment/self-criticism
- ignoring your feelings by staying focused on your thoughts
- ignoring and numbing your feelings by turning to addictions
- making others responsible for your pain, joy, safety, and worth

I had been working with Randy for a few weeks when he said during a Skype session, "I don't understand why bad things keep happening to me. It's been one thing after another with employees quitting and other bad stuff with my business and problems with my family."

"Randy, what are you feeling right now?"

"Anxious. I'm always anxious."

"Are you willing to take responsibility for what you are telling yourself that is causing your anxiety?"

"Yes, at least I think I am."

"Ask your inner child — your feeling self, your soul essence — what you are telling yourself right now or what you are doing or how you are treating yourself that is making you feel anxious."

"I think I'm always telling myself that I'm never good enough, that I haven't accomplished enough, that I'm not conscious enough, that I will never get this. It seems to me that this is background noise for me, that I'm always telling myself things like this."

"Why?"

Randy pauses for a moment: "I'm not sure. I think it has something to do with being okay only when I accomplish things. There are always things that need to get done."

"So is your worth tied up in getting things done, in accomplishing things?"

"Yes."

"Do you believe that you need to judge yourself to motivate yourself to get things done?"

"Yes, I think that is exactly what's happening."

"So according to your wounded self, you have no intrinsic worth; your worth and identity are in your accomplishments?"

"I don't know anything about my intrinsic worth. How would I know about that?"

In a previous session, I had helped Randy connect with his Divine guidance. He named his guidance Luke. Since Randy was currently open to learning and he had been eating well since we started our sessions, he was able to connect.

"Randy, ask Luke to show you what he sees when he looks at you as a little boy, who you really are."

Randy paused, tuned in, and quietly stated: "I was a sweet and happy little boy, kind and caring with others."

"Is there anything wrong with this little boy — anything about him that isn't okay, isn't lovable?"

"No, he's wonderful." Tears welled up in Randy's eyes.

"This is your essence, who you really are — your intrinsic worth. And this little boy within you, your core self, is letting you know that by being anxious, you are not seeing yourself and you are rejecting yourself with all your self-judgments. As long as you judge yourself and create an ongoing anxiety, your vibrancy is too low to manifest what you want. In fact, you may be drawing to you what you don't want instead of what you do want."

"As I'm thinking about this, I realize it's not just me that I judge. I judge everyone. It's ongoing in my head — either judging myself or judging others. I think I really am addicted to judgment."

"Yes, and what do you think the judgment is protecting you from feeling?"

"Oh, now that you ask, I know exactly what it's protecting me from. It's what we were talking about in the last session about my childhood. I'm protecting myself from the loneliness I've always felt and the helplessness over the pain of my childhood. Hmm. I wonder whether I've always preferred the anxiety to the loneliness and heart-break of my childhood."

"That's likely true because the anxiety is something you can control with your judgments, so it covers your feelings of helplessness concerning others. Are you ready to feel these painful feelings now that you are an adult? Are you ready to bring in your loving Divine guidance to help you finally feel and heal these feelings so that you don't need to use judgment to avoid them? Are you ready to stop rejecting and abandoning yourself?"

"Yes, I'm more than ready!"

Moving out of self-judgment and into self-compassion and

self-forgiveness takes much consciousness — much awareness and mindfulness. Most of us have been judging ourselves and others for so long that it has become automatic. It takes much consciousness to move into compassion and acceptance for ourselves and others, but with practice, we can move out of abandoning ourselves and into being loving to ourselves.

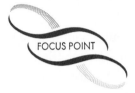

FOCUS POINT

Most of us have been judging ourselves and others for so long that it has become automatic. It takes much consciousness to move into compassion and acceptance for ourselves and others.

Thoughts That Create Stress

A major way we emotionally abandon ourselves is by stressing ourselves out with our thoughts. Staying healthy is a three-pronged endeavor involving food, exercise, and state of mind. A good state of mind is most important for good health — more important even than genes, food, or exercise — with the way we handle stress emerging as a major player. It not only directly influences health factors such as our blood pressure but also figures in to why we indulge in poor eating habits. Food and beverages as well as other addictions become a means of relieving our stress, at least in the short term.

We become stressed for a variety of reasons, ranging from the effect of some of the foods we ingest to lack of physical activity, schedules that are far too hectic, and the impact of painful events. And as I discussed in the last chapter, self-rejection and various forms of emotional self-abandonment are major causes of stress.

One of the most important regulatory mechanisms with which the human body is equipped is the autonomic nervous system. Designed to enable us to mobilize when necessary, this system is known as the fight-or-flight mechanism. In addition to thrusting us into an energized mode to be prepared to either confront danger or run from it, the autonomic nervous system can also put us into a freeze condition akin to that of a rabbit or deer caught in headlights.

During the eons when our species was evolving on the African plains and in rain forests and jungles, we were potential prey for hungry lions or crocodiles. The fight-or-flight response developed because we needed to be able to spring into defensive action at a moment's notice.

Although for much of our time on the planet this ability to summon instant strength was crucial for our survival, most of us no longer have to contend with ravenous big cats or crocodiles intent on ingesting us for dinner. Nevertheless, the mechanism that evolved to allow us to cope with such dangers is still very much a part of how the human body functions.

Many aspects of modern life stress us. For young people in school, bullying is a major threat, activating not only the fight-or-flight mechanism but frequently also the freeze response. A phone call from a debt collection agency brings a specific reaction in most of us, and even receiving our electricity bill or bank statement can trigger us, setting off a sense of panic.

If we find ourselves being attacked physically, the protective mechanism we refer to as the stress response springs into action. In a flash, the body focuses on channeling maximum energy to those parts that are adapted to self-protection, especially our extremities, automatically drawing blood from our organs and using it to bolster the supply to our arms and legs so that we can either do battle or run. Thus, whenever the part of the brain geared to our survival is activated, several of our organs are robbed of necessary nutrients, which means our immune systems aren't functioning at an optimum level.

Once the danger has passed and we've discharged the chemicals involved in our response by either fighting or making a quick getaway, our bodies return to equilibrium. Blood again flows to our organs and immune systems in an optimum way. So finely tuned is our autonomic nervous system that it doesn't take the imminence of a car crash, being taunted by a bully, or being pursued by a debt collector or potential attacker to trigger it. All that's needed is for us to *believe* we are in danger, even when our actual survival isn't in question.

In so many cases in modern life, it's our thoughts that generate our stress. Via the news, we hear about someone being attacked and then imagine being attacked ourselves. Or we imagine being rejected, running out of money, being fired from our jobs, or losing a loved one. The body goes into the stress response the moment we begin thinking scary thoughts. In such a situation, there's no actual physical danger requiring a response from the autonomic nervous system. The problem is that *the body doesn't know the difference between something that's really happening and what's transpiring only in our heads.*

One of the most important steps any of us can take to improve our health and well-being is to become aware of when our thoughts are generating stress. Once we do so, we can learn how to alter that state of mind, eventually becoming adept at arresting stressful thinking. It's for this reason that people who have learned the art of letting challenging situations roll off their backs tend to enjoy better health than others.

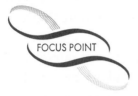

FOCUS POINT

Become aware of when your thoughts generate stress so that you can alter your state of mind and eventually arrest stressful thinking.

The damaging thing about thoughts that trigger our stress response is that instead of burning up the chemicals that fuel our ability to fight or flee, we're stuck with them flooding our systems. Because there's no physical release, the stress caused by our thoughts lacks an off switch. Strenuous exercise might help dissipate the charged state we are in, but if we keep thinking scary thoughts, the stress will come right back. The state of being stuck in this cycle is what we experience as anxiety.

This is the problem with the third aspect of the stress response, which is when we freeze. In this case, there could be real and present danger, but we are in a situation in which we are unable to fight or flee. We are rendered helpless in a form of dissociation. This makes us prisoners of the negative effects of the chemical reactions taking place in our bodies because (as with the fight-or-flight response) when it results from our imaginations, we don't get to fight or run, thereby discharging the energy.

If we were physically or sexually abused as children, we might have dissociated as a way of managing the abuse. We might have dissociated to such an extent that we don't remember the abuse. If the abuse we suffered was extreme enough, we might have become fragmented as a person so that parts of ourselves don't relate to other parts, and each part handles only an aspect of the abuse. This is what happens when people experience what we used to call multiple personality disorder (MPD) and now is called dissociative identity disorder (DID). We now know that this is a brilliant, life-saving coping strategy for surviving the unbearable.

Whenever we end up stuck in a fearful state, it can erode our health and certainly lower our vibrancy and our ability to connect with our Divine guidance. To allow the challenges of life to constantly stress us is to invite health problems. Even if we eat well and engage in adequate exercise, allowing ourselves to entertain the kind of thoughts that precipitate stress constitutes a form of self-rejection. We are, in effect, abandoning ourselves — though, now that we are adults, quite unnecessarily.

Imagine telling a child the kinds of things we tell ourselves that cause stress. Wouldn't that child feel frightened, alone, or abandoned? It's no different for us as adults when we tell ourselves we "can't handle" being rejected or being alone. We're bound to feel anxious. If we imagine this is "killing us," which is so often our response to some kind of actual or perceived slight, it will gradually do just that.

Yet the fact is that we are not being honest with ourselves. As adults, we can learn to manage life's challenges, and we can learn to release old trauma from our bodies. Fortunately today there are numerous trauma therapies to help us "unfreeze" and release trapped energy.[1]

When you were a child, it is true that you could have died if you were left alone. But unless you are ill, old, or disabled, it isn't true of you as an adult. Instead of paying attention to your programmed ego mind, which developed all kinds of fears in childhood and can easily scare you if you have never let go of those fears, you can listen for the inner knowing that says, "I can handle rejection. I've been rejected

---

1.   See Dr. David Berceli's book and DVD *The Revolutionary Trauma Process*, both from Namaste Publishing. Also review the work of the Somatic Experiencing Trauma Institute and Dr. Peter Levine's bestselling *Waking the Tiger: Healing Trauma*. Additionally, the Emotional Freedom Technique (EFT) has proved valuable to many. See http://www.EmoFree.com, or perform an Internet search to discover other websites that feature EFT.

many times, and it didn't kill me. I've been alone many times, and I didn't die." When you tell yourself the truth, your body will release the anxiety, and you will feel peaceful. Your peaceful feeling is telling you that you are now thinking the truth.

This might surprise you, but anxiety isn't an enemy to be conquered. Rather, it's a teacher we need to heed. Whenever you feel anxious, your autonomic nervous system is letting you know that you're buying into a thought that's untrue, and thoughts that are repeated become beliefs. Our false beliefs are lies we have repeated and now cause us unnecessary physical stress and limitation.

We know a belief is false when the belief itself causes us fear, anxiety, depression, shame, guilt, anger, or a feeling of emptiness and inner aloneness. We then make the mistake of trying to protect against the pain caused by our false beliefs by sinking into various addictions and other ways of controlling ourselves and others.

Instead of trying to get rid of these painful feelings, try learning from them by asking yourself, "What am I telling myself that's causing me to feel anxious, depressed, shamed, guilty, angry, or empty? What untrue thoughts from my wounded ego are scaring me or hurting me?" This is the way you can become aware of the old, programmed, false beliefs you might have absorbed in childhood that are limiting you and causing you stress now.

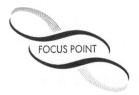

FOCUS POINT

Instead of trying to get rid of painful feelings, try learning from them by asking yourself probing questions.

Relational Self-Abandonment

You already know that the primary ways we physically abandon ourselves is with junk food, alcohol, drugs, and lack of exercise, as well as with not getting enough sleep. How do you abandon yourself in relationships? Do the following statements apply to you?

- I give myself up, going along with what the other person wants so that I gain that person's approval and avoid his or her disapproval, anger, or rejection.
- I shut down and withdraw rather than speak my truth.

- I avoid advocating for myself in the face of others' angry, blaming, invasive, or disrespectful behavior toward me.
- I allow others to emotionally, physically, or sexually abuse me.
- I become angry and blame others when they don't take care of me in the ways I want.
- I make others' feelings and needs more important than mine and take care of others' feelings and needs while ignoring mine.
- I agree with others even when I disagree, compromising my integrity.
- I judge my feelings, looking to others to validate them for me.
- I ignore my existential painful feelings of loneliness, heartbreak, sorrow, grief, or helplessness over others and instead pretend that I am okay.
- I have sex when I don't want to in order to avoid my partner's anger or rejection.
- I resist others out of fear of being controlled, even not doing things I actually want to do.

What else might you do to compromise your integrity and make you feel alone, anxious, and abandoned? When we are filled with painful feelings and are not open to Divine guidance to help us learn from and release them, we might dump them on others in various ways in an effort to release them. How do you dump your feelings on others? Here are some common responses.

- **I yell at, judge, or blame others**, hoping they will do one of three things: understand how much I'm hurting and change what they are doing; be compassionate, caring, and approving; or give me permission to do something I want to do but am not allowing myself to do.
- **I calmly and relentlessly complain** about something over and over, badgering others with the hope that they will say just the right thing to release the painful feelings in me. I believe that if they agree, change, or acknowledge what they are doing, I will feel better. Even if they do say the right thing, I keep at it, because it's never right enough.
- **I cry as a pathetic victim**, hoping others will feel badly enough to give me the compassion I'm not giving myself or will stop doing what they are doing that is hurting me so that I don't have to take loving action for myself.

- **I talk on and on**, addictively, hoping that if I talk enough and get enough attention from others, my pain will release.
- **I shut down and withdraw my love** from others, hoping they will feel badly enough to change and give me the understanding and compassion I'm not giving to myself.
- **I try to have sex** with my partner to release my stress and validate myself.

What happens in your relationships when you behave in any of these addictive ways? Is your relationship thriving or falling apart because of your self-abandonment? While these wounded, self-abandoning behaviors work temporarily to distract you from your pain, they all result in more disconnection and loneliness between you and those important to you, as well as disconnection from your Divine guidance. While it might seem as if the pain subsides when you dump your feelings on others, all that really happens is that the feelings go deeper and get stuck in your body, perhaps even causing physical problems.

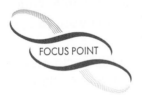

FOCUS POINT

While wounded, self-abandoning behaviors may work temporarily to distract you from your pain, they result in more disconnection and loneliness.

Spiritual Self-Abandonment

We spiritually abandon ourselves when we turn to externals to fill inner emptiness rather than turning to our Divine guidance. How do you spiritually abandon yourself? Consider these statements:

- When I feel alone and empty, I turn to substance or process addictions to fill up.
- I make others or my partner into my higher power by expecting him or her to be my dependable source of love.
- I never dialogue with Divine guidance.
- My thoughts and actions are not governed by my guidance. Instead, they are governed by my ego.
- I rarely feel grateful for what I have, the beauty of nature, or the love I experience.

- I don't let go and let God. I don't surrender outcomes to Spirit. Instead, I try to play God and control the outcomes.
- I don't pray or meditate.
- I don't have a spiritual community of like-minded people to support me.
- I don't attend to what has heart and meaning for me. I don't listen to my soul regarding my path.
- I don't help others, nor do I do any service for others.
- Love, truth, and kindness are not my guiding lights. I'm more guided by controlling time, money, people, and outcomes.

A personal experience of Divine love is available to each of us, so why don't more of us turn to this experience? Why do we turn to food, sex, TV, work, drugs, alcohol — almost anything — rather than fill our emptiness with the love and grace of our Divine guidance? The sad answer is that the spiritual abuse in our homes, churches, and schools could be in the way of our experiencing a direct, personal experience of God as divine love and wisdom. If you were raised in a Judeo-Christian religion, perhaps you were taught the following:

- God is judgmental and controlling, and you don't want to open to a judgmental, controlling God.
- God is an old man in the sky who, like Santa Claus, "knows when you've been bad or good," so "you'd better watch out." (This is not a very appealing concept of God or of Santa Claus.)
- God doesn't exist, and anyone who believes in God is using God as a crutch.
- What if people are wrong about the existence of God? You don't want to risk being duped and looking stupid.
- Only special people have a direct line to God. You can't trust your own experience. You need to trust your religious or spiritual leader.
- You don't deserve God's love. God is there for others but not for you.
- You were born in sin, and you need to spend your life proving your worth to be loved by God.
- You can't expect God to care about you and answer your prayers. God is too busy.

I am often asked by my clients, "If God is all-powerful, why didn't he stop my father" (or mother, brother, babysitter, uncle, or a stranger) "from abusing me? Why does he allow all this abuse to go on?" This question indicates that the person does not understand what God is. Were you programmed to believe that God is a person in the sky who can stop people from doing awful things rather than the spirit of love, compassion, wisdom, and joy? Even the Bible states that "God is Spirit" (John 4:24, ESV) and "God is love" (1 John 4:8, ESV).

Since we all have free will, we all decide when to open or close our hearts. God cannot enter a closed heart. God comes into our hearts by invitation, and we invite God into our hearts when our intention is to love ourselves and others.

Abusers have closed their hearts to God. Their intention is to protect themselves against their own pain. God cannot guide them because their hearts are closed. When people close their hearts, they cut off their empathy and compassion. They stop caring about the effect they have on others and can therefore do untold harm. Very likely, their parents or caregivers had closed their hearts, and if they were abused or didn't receive the love they needed, they learned to do the same thing in trying to manage the pain. The result is that they may do to others what was done to them. The legacy of abuse is very sad.

Financial Self-Abandonment

Did you grow up in a family that demonstrated personal responsibility for financial safety, or did one or both of your parents or other caregivers demonstrate self-abandonment in this important area? What do you do that creates financial stress for you? These are all forms of financial self-abandonment, and they all cause stress.

- I have major credit card debt and pay high interest.
- My bills are greater than my income.
- I use spending as an addictive way to self-soothe.
- I am growing older with little or no retirement money set aside.
- I have no idea where all my money goes because I don't keep track.
- I have lots of investments and plenty of income, but I am still anxious about money.
- I try to control my partner regarding money even when there is plenty.

- I deprive myself of vacations or other things I want even when there is enough money.
- My identity or sense of worth is attached to how much money I have.
- I am a physically healthy adult capable of working and do not have small children at home, but I am dependent on someone else for my financial safety.

Do you have a spending addiction or a shopping addiction? Do you rush out to buy things when you feel stressed? Do you have to have the best of everything — the best shoes, the best car, the best house? Do you max out your credit cards? Do you live in fear that your partner or your parents — whomever you are financially dependent on — will cut you off from their financial support? Do you refuse to get professional training so that you can earn your own money, even in the face of this threat?

If you relate to any of these, you are abandoning yourself financially. The message to yourself when you financially abandon yourself, as with all forms of self-abandonment, is that you are not worthy enough to have financial safety or that you are not worthy enough to enjoy the money you have earned.

If you are tying your self-worth to money, then you will likely never feel happy, peaceful, worthy, or safe because self-worth has to do with loving and valuing who you really are and how you treat yourself rather than with anything external.

Organizational Self-Abandonment

Organizational responsibility concerns how we manage our time and space. You are abandoning yourself and not taking organizational responsibility regarding time when you do the following:
- often rush to get things done
- often are late to appointments
- rarely have time for yourself
- have no balance between work and play
- don't have much time for family and friends
- often feel overwhelmed and anxious regarding getting things done
- tend to procrastinate
- generally pay bills and taxes late

- can't find the time to respond to emails in a timely fashion
- can't find the time to cook healthy food
- can't find the time to exercise or get enough sleep

You are not taking organizational responsibility regarding space when you do the following:
- often can't find what you are looking for
- create clutter by having papers, mail, magazines, and other items stacked up in piles or scattered in disarray
- still have things packed in boxes or not put away from the last time you moved
- have not created a peaceful and aesthetically pleasing environment in your work and home spaces

Taking organizational responsibility is part of taking emotional responsibility. It's part of lowering your stress level. All forms of self-abandonment create stress, which lowers your vibrancy and makes it very difficult to connect with your Divine guidance. Vibrancy results from eating the way your body needs to eat and loving yourself the way your core self needs to be loved.

Resistance Is a Major Form of Self-Abandonment

To eat well and take care of our health in other ways requires a certain amount of organization. We can't just stop at a fast-food joint for lunch or pick up a frozen dinner on our way home from work. We have to think ahead and do a little planning. A lack of forethought, planning, and organization will not only torpedo a desire to eat healthily but also introduce additional stress, which is itself detrimental to health.

If we wish to feel in tiptop condition, it's essential to address the stress we create when we are in a state of disarray instead of being organized. This stress is caused directly by our disorganized state and indirectly by the effect it has on how we tend to skimp on eating well and in a relaxed manner when our lives are in chaos.

You might be thinking, "It's all well and good to say I need to be more organized. I already know this, but I can't seem to do anything about it. I'm stuck in this area. What can I do to change things?"

We touched on the urge to resist being controlled in the previous chapter. Now we need to look at it in a different context. When resisting being controlled is more important than loving yourself, you will remain stuck in your disorganized state.

The adolescent part of us is often resistant to being controlled, even by ourselves. "You can't tell me what to do" is the refrain of the adolescent, which in turn is a recapitulation of being a two-year-old. The wounded adolescent part of us gets a grim type of pleasure out of resisting control. It likes to believe we can get away with things and derives a dark satisfaction from doing as little as we can, especially if we can get someone to do it for us.

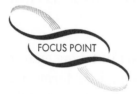

FOCUS POINT

When resisting being controlled is more important than loving yourself, you will remain stuck in your disorganized state.

What limiting beliefs from your ego might you be operating from that keep you resistant? Let's look at some common beliefs:

Resisting control is essential to my integrity and individuality. This might have been true when you were a child. As an adult, integrity and individuality come from making your own decisions based on what's best for you rather than basing your decisions on avoiding being controlled. When you make decisions regarding what's best for you, you come from your personal power.

Resisting control establishes my independent identity. As a child, this might have been true, but as an adult, your identity lies in making your own choices, independent of whether another is trying to control you.

My only option when another person is attempting to control me is to comply or to resist. This is the only option for your wounded self. But when your core self and Divine guidance guide you, your actions come from your desire to be the loving person you really are.

I am really being my own person when I resist. When you resist, you might not realize that your resistance is controlling you. All another person has to do to have control over you is to demand something from you, and your behavior will be determined by your reaction rather than your desires. When your goal is to resist being controlled, you must resist, which means you no longer have free choice. You are being your own person only when you decide that loving yourself is more important to you than resisting control.

It's the controlling person's fault that I resist. Your wounded self might argue that if the other person wasn't so controlling, you wouldn't have to resist. However, to resist is your choice and has nothing to do with someone trying to control you. You always have the option of learning about what loving yourself would actually mean.

If I didn't resist, I'd be swallowed up. This might have been true for you as a child, but as an adult, you can learn to set loving boundaries rather than resist.

The sad thing is that the grim pleasure and dark satisfaction of resisting control or getting away with things can't hold a candle to the peace and joy of taking loving care of ourselves. The ego wounded self, which constantly lies to us, can't see that by resisting responsibility, we are deeply limiting our ability to manifest our creativity, thereby denying ourselves the profound satisfaction that comes from expressing who we truly are.

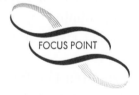

FOCUS POINT

The grim pleasure of resisting control or getting away with things can't hold a candle to the peace and joy of taking loving care of ourselves.

All this changes when our intent changes. By making the decision that loving ourselves is more important than abandoning ourselves by resisting control and getting away with things, we move out of the wounded adolescent state and into the loving adult state. Do you see why so many of us refuse to eat the way we know is in our highest good or exercise to promote health and in other ways allow behavior detrimental to our health to slip by us against our better judgment?

So many clients have told me, "But I just don't have time to shop for organic foods and then go home and prepare them. I constantly run late. I'm so rushed off my feet that I barely have time to stick a pizza in the oven for dinner." Many of us feel too rushed to spend time carefully selecting and preparing what we eat. Joe is an example, having grown up with a mother who was always rushing him.

From the time Joe was a child, his mother would become angry with him if he wasn't ready to leave on time. But it wasn't just dawdling that Joe was punished for. Joe's mother wanted control over just about everything regarding her son — the clothes he wore, the friends he chose, and how he spent his time. Being a good boy, Joe gave in, except when it came to being on time. This became his way of taking a stand, his means of resisting his mother's total control of him.

As an adult, Joe still has problems being on time. He's late for doctors' appointments, meetings at work, movies and plays, and getting home, and he has no time to spend with his family. Because he resists managing his time, he ends up grabbing fast food for lunch and often for dinner. As for exercise, when is he supposed to fit that in?

No matter how upset or angry his wife and children are over his lateness, nothing budges his determination to be consistently late. Even the fact that he's upset with himself because he knows he's harming his health by eating junk and failing to work out has zero impact. Does this sound like you or someone you know?

If you are going to take good care of your health, being able to organize your time is a must. Otherwise, you'll take the easy route of dropping into a fast-food joint or loading your shopping cart with packaged meals as you rush along the supermarket aisles on your dash home from work.

When Joe started working with me, he was often late for his appointments and each time felt it necessary to explain, apologize, and defend himself as if I must be upset with him. I clarified that it was his time he was depriving himself of since he was paying for it even when he showed up late. In fact, I didn't mind the five or ten minutes of paid vacation! When Joe finally got that I had no expectation or concern regarding when he arrived for his appointment, he had nothing left to rebel against except himself. Because he liked working with me, from then on, he was more often on time.

CHAPTER 12

YOU CAN CHANGE YOUR BRAIN

Daniel Siegel, MD, says, "becoming open to our body's states — the feelings in our heart, the sensations in our belly, the rhythm of our breathing — is a powerful source of knowledge.... Bringing our sensations into awareness enables intuition to blossom and sometimes can offer lifesaving information."[1] If we are going to kick the junk food habit, along with any other poor eating habits that might not only be affecting our health but also limiting our ability to enjoy a life-changing spiritual connectedness, it's necessary to change our thinking about food and health in general. The old brain patterns, such as my addiction to sugar in my earlier life, have to go.

It used to be believed we couldn't change our brain patterns and that as neurons die new ones are not created. With the advent of MRIs, brain research has shown this to be untrue. We now know that thousands of new neurons are created daily through a process called

---

1.   Daniel Siegel, MD, *Mindsight* (New York: Bantam, 2010) p. 63.

neurogenesis — a process that enables us to change our mental and emotional habits to a remarkable degree.

Whether the new neurons formed in our brains each day live or die depends on whether we engage in effortful learning. It turns out that what we focus on is what gets programmed into the brain since the process of focusing creates new neural pathways. The implications for our dietary and emotional habits and overall health are enormous.

I have been able to validate this research in my life. I'm very different from the person I was before I started to connect with my core self and my Divine guidance. In fact, long before the current brain research validated my experience — and that of many of my clients — I knew that my brain was being rewired through the Inner Bonding practice of self-love, resulting not only in inner peace, joy, and Divine connection but also in the ability to love others.

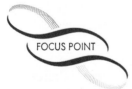

FOCUS POINT

What we focus on is what gets programmed into the brain since the process of focusing creates new neural pathways.

Healing Is Always Possible

You may be wondering whether those who were seriously damaged by their upbringing are beyond hope of recovery. I am aware of the research that indicates how infants and toddlers who don't receive adequate love, along with help learning self-regulation, fail to develop the part of their brains responsible for regulating their feelings.[2] The first two years of a child's life are crucial to the development of this dimension of the brain. However, my experience with clients has taught me that it's never too late to accomplish huge change, no matter what happened during those formative years.

As I mentioned, my brain has changed, as have the brains of many who have sought my help. Of course, it would be much easier on all of us had we developed this capacity in the first two years of our lives.

---

2. Sue Gerhardt, *Why Love Matters* (Abingdon United Kingdom: Routledge, 2014) pp. 18–19.

But if this didn't happen for you, be assured that you can learn to do this yourself.

As your true self enters the picture and you develop your loving adult through your Divine connection, taking loving action for yourself, your brain will rewire itself, enabling you to tap into your capacity for self-regulation. You'll be able to walk down the supermarket aisles and pick out the foods that truly feed your body and mind, passing up the endless forms of packaged dead concoctions that can't possibly enliven your cells. You'll drink only a celebratory glass of wine instead of a whole bottle. You'll spend extra to shop at stores that carry organic foods instead of junk, realizing this is a small investment in your health compared to the cost of fixing a serious illness later. You'll take time to prepare healthful meals for your family — and equally so for yourself if you're single, since no one is as important in your life as you are.

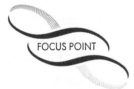

FOCUS POINT

As your true self enters the picture and you develop your loving adult through your Divine connection, you brain will rewire itself.

Consistent practice rewires the brain and frees us from the false beliefs that, as we touched on earlier, are often a major cause of anxiety, depression, guilt, shame, anger, addictions, aloneness, emptiness, and relationship problems. The deep programming in the lower brain — the amygdala, which is the home of the ego, the false wounded self — is gradually replaced by new wiring in the higher brain, the prefrontal cortex.

This rewiring eventually results in moving from fear into a sense of inner safety, from self-loathing to self-love, and from emptiness to feeling a fundamental oneness with everyone and everything. Instead of operating in the world as an ego, you begin operating as a powerful, spiritually connected, loving adult.

Given this understanding of the brain's plasticity, we can understand why Alfred Binet, the developer of the IQ test, stated, "With practice, training, and above all, method, we manage to increase our attention, our memory, our judgment and literally to become more intelligent than we were before."[3] If you were brought up to believe that a person's intelligence is fixed and can't be elevated, this is good news indeed. The same is true of our imaginations and creativity, both of which can flourish as new neural circuits are developed.

Of equal if not greater importance, our emotional intelligence can also be improved. If you tend to flare with anger, shoot your mouth off, indulge in episodes of envy or jealousy, or experience bouts of pouting and sulking, realize that your essential self is the source of none of these reactive emotions. They are the result of neural pathways developed in childhood, and they constitute learned behaviors that *can be unlearned.*

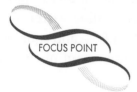

FOCUS POINT

Our emotional intelligence can be improved. Realize that your essential self is the source of none of you negative reactive emotions. They are the result of neural pathways developed in childhood, and they can be unlearned.

You've heard the adage, "You're never too old to learn." It turns out that is true. As Dr. Daniel Siegel points out, "Neuroplasticity is possible throughout the lifespan, not just in childhood." Like others, Siegel affirms that "the brain changes physically in response to experience, and new mental skills can be acquired with intentional effort, focused awareness, and concentration."[4]

One of the ways we can exercise focused awareness and exert intentional effort is explained by Jeffrey M. Schwartz, MD, and Rebecca Gladding, MD, who assert, "Refocusing on healthy, adaptive activities is what changes your brain in positive ways." These authors stress that "how you act and what you focus on shapes your brain in powerful ways."[5] It's this ability of the brain to change its way of

3. Robert J. Sternberg and Scott Barry Kaufman, *The Cambridge Handbook of Intelligence* (Cambridge University Press: 2011) p. 749.

4. Daniel Siegel, MD, *Mindsight* (New York: Bantam, 2010) p. 84.

5. Schwartz and Gladding, *You Are Not Your Brain* (New York: Avery Publishing, 2012) pp. 242-243. Jeffrey M. Schwartz, MD, is a research psychiatrist at the UCLA School of Medicine and a seminal thinker in the field of self-directed neuroplasticity, and Rebecca Gladding, MD, is a clinical instructor and attending psychiatrist at the UCLA Stewart and Lynda Resnick Neuropsychiatric Hospital and the Semel Institute for Neuroscience and Human Behavior.

functioning that can empower us to move from eating, thinking, and behaving in ways that harm us to eating, thinking, and behaving in ways that benefit us.

Spiritual connection involves being fully grounded in the body, which is a powerful antidote to detrimental habit patterns such as reaching for packaged nonfoods or stopping for fast food. The more in tune you are with your body, the less you'll gravitate to unhealthy eating practices.

The antithesis of a spiritually connected state is an anxious state. Whenever you feel anything less than peaceful and full, rather than either wallowing in it or fighting it, switch your focus to your body, and compassionately embrace your feelings. When we are connected to the body, allowing ourselves to fully inhabit it through breathing consciously and sinking deeply into it, we are far less likely to criticize ourselves and resort to our addictions (such as reaching for a drink or junk) or make someone else responsible for our disturbed state.

When many of us come to a point in our lives that to be spiritually connected is important to us, unfortunately we tend to do just the opposite of embracing our bodily state. Fantasizing that spirituality is something other than a way of experiencing our normal, everyday routine, we divorce the secular from the spiritual, often wishing we could just meditate all day in an ashram or something of the kind. Schwartz and Gladding correct this misguided notion by pointing out that it's refocusing on healthy, adaptive activities that changes us.[6] This is something we do as part of our normal routine by changing how we regard our bodies and our minds. To promote the vitality of both is essential in advancing our spiritual connection and thus our personal growth. A healthy food-and-thought diet does just that, whereas junk foods and junk thoughts keep us disconnected from ourselves and our Divine connection.

Because many of us were messed up by how we were raised, the strategies we resorted to were necessary to protect us from the over-whelming pain in our lives — the loneliness, heartbreak, and helplessness of childhood. However, we are each capable of moving beyond the

---

6. Schwartz and Gladding, *You Are Not Your Brain* (New York: Avery Publishing, 2012) pp. 242-243.

pain and jettisoning those strategies that don't befit a grown person. As Schwartz and Gladding state, "The less attention you pay to something (either with your thoughts or through your actions), the weaker the brain circuits associated with that sensation or action become."[7]

We can move forward in our growth, adapting to situations as they are now instead of being stuck in the past, by learning to constructively and lovingly manage whatever life sends our way. My experience, as well as that of countless clients, has taught me that the more we practice loving actions guided by our authentic, wise selves, the more these positive patterns of thinking and acting become ingrained in our brains.

Whereas I was once addicted to food and anger as I fulfilled the role as the caretaker of others while ignoring myself, I no longer suffer from these addictions. Whereas I used to react to others' anger and blame, I no longer defend or explain in an attempt to control how they feel about me, nor do I give myself up. Whereas I used to feel I wasn't good enough, I now cherish my true self and am highly motivated to take loving care of myself. Whereas I was focused on getting love, now I receive great joy from giving and sharing love out of a sense of my own fullness instead of based on neediness. I have guided many clients through a similar retooling of their lives.

The Importance of Mindfulness

We call the state in which "nothing goes unnoticed" mindfulness. In a study on mindfulness conducted at Harvard University (in this case centered on the effects of meditation), MRIs of the brain were administered to sixteen participants two weeks before the study and again after the eight weeks of the study. The images revealed "increased grey-matter density in the hippocampus, known to be important for learning and memory, and in structures associated with self-awareness, compassion and introspection."[8]

This particular study involved thirty minutes of meditation each

---

7. Schwartz and Gladding, *You Are Not Your Brain* (New York: Avery Publishing, 2012) p. 315.
8. Learn the details of this study at https://news.harvard.edu/gazette/story/2011/01/eight-weeks-to-a-better-brain/.

day with an emphasis on participants becoming aware of sensations, feelings, and their states of mind. Following the eight weeks, the participants reported reductions in stress paralleling the decrease of gray-matter density in the amygdala, which is known to play an important role in stress and anxiety.

Less stress coupled with greater compassion for ourselves, combined with less anxiety and increased awareness, affects another aspect of our lives that has a tremendous effect on our health and wellness — our relationships. A stressful relationship, particularly one laced with anger and accompanying feelings of loneliness, can bring on a heart attack, a stroke, debilitating back pain, headaches, and a host of other symptoms — along with driving us to feed our addictions to food, excessive alcohol, smoking, pharmaceuticals, or illicit drugs.

Dr. Amy Banks, MD, (an instructor in psychiatry at Harvard Medical School and now the director of Advanced Training at the Jean Baker Miller Training Institute at the Wellesley Centers for Women) asks, "So, what does your brain have to do with relationships? The answer is, well, everything. Science has shown that specific neural pathways exist to actively help us engage in healthy relationships, and that in healthy relationships, those pathways grow stronger and stronger." Sadly the opposite is also true: "In chronic bad relationships, these pathways do not get the extra stimulation they need. These neural pathways actually get weaker, and so do your relationships."[9]

The book you are holding in your hands addresses self-healing on the physical, emotional, relational, and spiritual levels. You've seen how we learned to reject and abandon ourselves and the impact this has had on both body and mind. Now that you know you can change your patterns of rejecting and abandoning yourself, walk with me through a profound self-healing process that will facilitate a powerful spiritual connection to the whole of reality.

---

9. You can read this article at https://www.mindbodygreen.com/0-17619/how-to-rewire-your-brain-for-stronger-relationships.html.

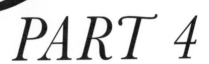

PART 4

ACTION: USE THE SIX STEPS TO INNER BONDING

Achieve At-Will Spiritual Connection
to Heal Yourself Physically, Emotionally,
and Spiritually

CHAPTER 13

INNER BONDING STEP 1: WILLINGNESS AND RESPONSIBILITY

We can't set out on a journey without the willingness to do so. Without the willingness to do whatever it takes to heal, we won't engage in the task of evolving our souls in the ability to love, which is essential for Divine connection. Along with high vibrancy through healthy eating, our vibrancy skyrockets when we are open to learning about loving ourselves and others.

The journey starts with step one of Inner Bonding: the willingness to feel pain and take responsibility for your feelings. This means choosing to become mindful of your feelings and being willing to take responsibility for the ways in which you might be causing your pain, for nurturing your existential pain, and for creating peace and joy for yourself.

Since one of the major ways our Divine guidance communicates with us is through our feelings, we are cutting off our guidance when we avoid experiencing our feelings. Therefore, we need to be willing to be present in our bodies with our feelings to be aware of our inner guidance.

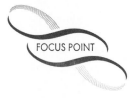

Divine guidance communicates with us through our feelings, so we need to be present in our body with our feelings to be aware of our inner guidance.

Willingness means we have decided to face our fears, our demons, the shadow side of ourselves — our wounded selves that most of us try to hide from everyone. It also means we are ready to stop hiding from ourselves so that we're no longer in denial about the pain we're in. We are ready to stop emotionally rejecting and abandoning ourselves by avoiding our feelings.

Willingness means being open to learning to move toward our feelings rather than away from them with our various addictions and other forms of self-abandonment. We learn to embrace them rather than ignore them.

Willingness involves doing whatever it takes, which means we're prepared to feel, understand, and take full responsibility for the whole range of our painful emotions — our wounded feelings of fear, anxiety, nervousness, blame, anger, irritation, impatience, hurt, shame, guilt, emptiness, aloneness, jealousy, and depression, along with our deeper existential feelings of loneliness, heartache, heartbreak, grief, sorrow, and helplessness concerning others. Willingness also means that we are ready to see how we are responsible for causing our wounded feelings by becoming aware of our thoughts, beliefs, and actions that are creating them.

When I tell people that they need to be willing to feel their pain, they often say to me, "What's the big deal about that? I feel my pain all the time." But there is a big difference between feeling pain and having the willingness to feel it in order to learn from it. There is no healing in just feeling and expressing our pain. We can cry and rage forever, but if we are not willing to take responsibility for our pain, we will likely be stuck with it.

Many people feel their feelings and wallow in them, and in some cases, they blame someone else for them. While others' unloving behaviors and challenging events can cause our loneliness, heartbreak, grief, and helplessness concerning those people, it is still our responsibility to lovingly manage these feelings. Blaming others only serves to keep us stuck in victim mode. When we feel grief over the loss of someone we love or heartbreak because someone we care about is being mean to us, we are still responsible for learning to lovingly manage the grief and heartbreak.

Our wounded feelings — other than the anxiety and depression triggered in our brains from a toxic gut — result from what we tell ourselves and how we treat ourselves. If we do not pay attention to our emotional pain, we will continue thinking and acting in ways that cause us pain. All our feelings have important information for us.

Ask yourself this: When you want to binge, eat sugar, drink alcohol, use drugs, smoke; blame, hit, appease, or resist someone; run away, turn on the TV, gamble, or shop; masturbate with pornography or demand sex from your partner; or compulsively act out in any way, what are you feeling? Are you turning to your addictions to distract you from your painful feelings? Are you willing to open to learning from these feelings instead of blocking them with addictive behavior? Are you willing to stop emotionally abandoning yourself by avoiding your feelings?

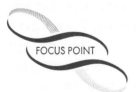

FOCUS POINT

If you do not pay attention to your emotional pain, you will continue to think and act in ways that cause your pain. Your feelings have important information for you.

Take Responsibility for Your Feelings

When we feel anything other than peace and fullness inside, the way forward is to decide that we *want* to take responsibility for our feelings because they have vital information for us. If we don't truly want to learn and take responsibility, we will automatically come from our egos and play the part of the victim. It requires a conscious decision to take responsibility for our feelings.

You can begin by saying to yourself, "I'm feeling bad" (or angry, jealous, impatient, and so forth), "and I want to take responsibility for causing this feeling." You might say, "I feel lonely and heartbroken, and I want to take responsibility for lovingly managing these emotions." The moment you experience a painful feeling or even minor unease, immediately say to yourself, "I want to take responsibility for this feeling." Try not to leave it for later — unless you are at work or in another situation where you can't immediately attend to your feelings.

When you feel wounded in some way, which could trigger any number of emotions ranging from anger to jealousy or anxiety, the wounded feeling might not be based on a present reality. The present situation could be evoking a false belief you absorbed in your past. Suppose that in your past, you were emotionally, physically, or sexually abused. Because you weren't at a place in life where you could understand that the abuse had nothing to do with anything you are or anything you did, only with the one inflicting it, you likely thought the abuse was your fault because you were not good enough. This became an ingrained belief you hold concerning yourself.

As an adult, when people are unloving to you, instead of feeling the deeper existential pain of the heartache, loneliness, and helplessness over their unloving behavior and thereby attending to your feelings with compassion for yourself, you might tell yourself they are being unloving because you aren't good enough or lovable enough or that you did something to cause them to be mean. Since you don't cause the abuser's unloving behavior, the hurt feelings that arise in you when you judge yourself aren't based in reality. They come from your false beliefs about yourself. Were your feelings based in reality, you would recognize that someone being mean isn't about you, and you would be very gentle with your heartache resulting from their unloving behavior.

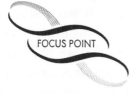

FOCUS POINT

Someone else's behavior toward you has nothing to do with you.

I'm not saying it's at all easy to manage some of the big challenges and tragedies you face in your life, but I've seen over and over how people who have strong, spiritually connected, loving adult selves bring sufficient love and compassion to their painful feelings to manage what life brings them.

Just as our wounded feelings come from our false beliefs and our resulting self-abandoning behavior, so do our addictions. This is why addictions gradually fall away once we learn to define our self-worth and love ourselves rather than continue to abandon ourselves. The more we open to learning about what our feelings are telling us and who we truly are and what loving ourselves looks like, the stronger our spiritual connection becomes.

The key is to recognize the difference between having the intention to protect, avoid, and control and having the intention to learn about loving ourselves. It's the intention to learn to love ourselves rather than continuing to abandon ourselves that opens the door to an ongoing, moment-by-moment consciousness of spiritual connection to and real-life experience of our oneness with the Divine. Along with eating very well, our intent to learn about loving ourselves is what raises our frequency high enough to connect with Divine guidance.

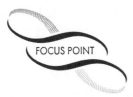

FOCUS POINT

The intent to learn to love ourselves, rather than continuing to abandon ourselves, opens the door to an ongoing, moment-by-moment consciousness of our spiritual connection to and real-life experience of our oneness with the Divine.

When Patty, a client, was aware of feeling bad, she would completely forget that her *thoughts* were causing her wounded feelings. When I felt she was ready, I asked her, "Are you willing to explore this?"

"I've been thinking about this," she confirmed. "When I was little, I wasn't allowed to express my feelings, or I would be punished. My parents had no empathy or compassion for my feelings. I decided that it was safer not to feel except when I was with someone who was compassionate toward me."

"I see," I said. "So are you making others responsible for whether or not you feel?"

"I think I believe it feels good only when someone else is compassionate toward me," Patty replied.

"So you either expend a lot of energy trying to get others to care about your feelings or just ignore your feelings and feel abandoned?"

Patty sighed. "It feels so good when someone else really gets me, really understands me."

"Have you ever really tried to get you?"

After a moment of thought, Patty answered, "I guess not."

"Obviously it has been a lifelong project of your wounded ego to garner empathy, compassion, and understanding from others, which is why you become irritated and at times angry when you don't get what you want."

Sighing again, Patty said, "I'm tired of being this way. After all, I have a great adult self in other areas of my life."

"Then how about asking your inner guidance whether it's truly better to seek love from someone else rather than showing it to yourself," I suggested.

Patty concluded she would feel much better if she took responsibility for loving herself. Realizing she would always feel desperate to be loved unless she took responsibility, she began shopping for nutritious food and preparing meals for herself. As she allowed the lonely feeling she at first experienced to simply be there instead of running from it or wallowing in it, she actually began to enjoy fixing healthy food.

The Fear of Feeling the Deep, Painful Feelings

With the advent of mass communication via cellphones and computers along with the social media these technologies spawn, you would think we would be more connected now than has been possible at any other time in history. However, for many of us, the opposite is true. On a surface level, we touch base, but authentic, deep, meaningful connection seems to elude us more than ever. Indeed, Twitter, Facebook, and a host of other social media sites have increasingly become tools for attacking as much as informing or connecting with each other, even leading to suicides that are broadcast live.

When we look closely, we realize that behind our surface connection with each another lurks a profound sense of aloneness and loneliness in our lives. When we avoid our feelings, we lose touch with our soul essence — our feeling selves. And it's because most of us don't know who we are (which is why so many of us are searching for ourselves, seeking the reason for being here) that we might have difficulty being alone. As a result of being disconnected from our feelings and therefore our Divine guidance, we might feel empty and lonely when we're by ourselves.

Likewise, the reason we connect on such a surface level in much of modern life is that we don't know how to connect with our essential selves. With our core lost to us, we are adrift on a vast sea of emotional isolation. Until we bond inwardly with our authentic selves and our Divine guidance, deep connection with others will remain a rare commodity. The loneliness of surface contact will rule.

Being alone when we'd rather not be is a fact of life. Loneliness is a major issue in modern society. As I stated previously, in my many years of working with people, I've seen over and over how every one of our addictions has its roots in our intent to avoid the pain of loneliness, along with the feelings of heartbreak, grief, and helplessness where others are concerned that accompany it. Even if we realize that our addictions to food, drugs, alcohol, gambling, TV, work, spending, and so on are ways of avoiding pain, in most cases, we are unaware of the deeper painful feelings we are trying to avoid.

Because loneliness is often tinged with helplessness where others are concerned, it can be hard to bear. We don't consciously connect how helpless with respect to others and ourselves we felt in infancy, but the loneliness and helplessness where others are concerned can trigger feelings of the times we were left alone to cry with no one responding. If our crying didn't bring the help we needed, there was nothing we could do. Had no one eventually come, we would have died.

Consequently, feelings of loneliness and helplessness over others are often associated with a fear of death. Even if help arrived, perhaps there was little love with it, creating an overwhelmingly confusing experience for the infant. This is why loneliness and helplessness with respect to others can trigger intense anxiety. They hark back to that time in your life when you may have shut down to your deep feeling center — your authentic self, which once knew what it was to enjoy a sense of oneness with everyone and everything.

Big painful feelings are too much for little bodies. As children, we had no way of regulating our big feelings. We needed our parents to do this for us by lovingly and compassionately holding us, letting us know we weren't alone and assuring us our feelings were acceptable. How many of us had parents who did this for us? How many of us had parents who knew how to manage and regulate their *own* big painful feelings?

As adults, if we open to our painful feelings with deep compassion and a desire to learn about what they are trying to tell us, we can release them. It's only because we couldn't handle such pain as children that we continue to avoid them, numbing them with pharmaceuticals or illegal drugs, drowning them in alcohol, and stuffing them down inside us by bingeing on sweets or other junk foods.

To fail to face and learn from our feelings as an adult constitutes an abandonment of ourselves, and we end up compounding the big feelings that reside within us, unresolved from childhood. Now we suffer not only the loneliness and helplessness we could do nothing about long ago but also the feelings of aloneness, emptiness, anxiety, or depression that come with self-abandonment, as well as the hangovers, the constant tiredness and washed-out feeling, and ultimately, the ill health that results from unhealthy emotions and the addictions we turn to.

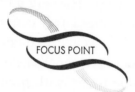

FOCUS POINT

Failing to learn from our feelings constitutes an abandonment of ourselves, and we end up compounding the big, unresolved feelings from childhood that reside within us.

While as children we could have died if left alone too long, this isn't true of us as adults. Instead of allowing our programmed minds to dominate — our wounded selves, which developed all kinds of fears and false beliefs in childhood and can easily scare us if we have never become aware of them — we can listen to what our feelings are telling us.

Once we become grounded in our loving essence and we take loving care of our feelings, the fact of being alone no longer feels threatening. After all, as I stated above, when we were small, had we been left alone, we would have died. It's not at all surprising that in times of loneliness, we often experience fear. When we were small, we were helpless over ourselves, but as adults, while we are still helpless where others are concerned, we are no longer helpless with respect to ourselves. We can feed ourselves or call for help.

However, as a result of ingrained patterns from our early days, as adults many of us choose not to embrace our power to take care of ourselves. Instead, we expend much energy avoiding our feelings — abandoning ourselves — and then trying to control others to get them to give us the love and attention we are not giving ourselves, which always proves to be a futile quest in the end.

The Challenge of Being Present with Your Feelings

Do you want to take responsibility for learning how you are creating your wounded feelings and for learning how to lovingly manage your deeper painful feelings? If you don't, then you might want to explore what is keeping you from accepting this responsibility. Are you deeply devoted to someone else taking away your pain and making you happy, believing that someone else can do it better than you? Are you afraid that you can't do it, that you are inadequate and can't learn to access your guidance and learn to take loving action? These are just two of the many false beliefs that might keep you stuck as a victim.

The idea of feeling your current or long-suppressed emotional pain might be very scary to you. Your fear of painful feelings is based on beliefs about pain that you acquired in childhood, beliefs that are false now that you are an adult. Let's review some of these false beliefs. See whether any of these ring a bell:

- My pain is too much for me. I'll go crazy or explode into a million pieces and die from it.
- If I open to my pain, it will be unending, a bottomless pit with no way out. It's better to keep a lid on it.
- There is no point in feeling my pain.
- No one wants to hear my pain. If I open to my pain, I will end up alone.
- Feeling and showing my pain is a sign of weakness and will lead to me being rejected.
- Feeling my pain makes me too vulnerable to being controlled by others.

To move beyond these false beliefs, you must be willing to test them and to prove them false. To test them, you must resist the urge to blunt your pain with substance and process addictions, such as staying in your head, judging yourself, or making others responsible for your feelings. You see, until you stop numbing yourself and avoiding your feelings in the face of your pain, you will never know that you can feel your pain without going crazy or dying. You will never know that your pain is not endless and that it can actually be a source of information and strength rather than weakness.

Some people have such deep pain from childhood abuse that they will not be able to endure opening to it until they have a solid, loving, spiritually connected adult in place. However, it is not advisable to attempt to open to the pain of severe abuse on your own. If you suspect that you might have deeply buried pain or trauma or if you have not succeeded in feeling your pain despite a genuine willingness to do so, it is imperative that you receive therapeutic help. Part of being a loving adult is asking for help when help is needed.

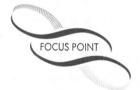

FOCUS POINT

Your pain is not endless, and it can actually be a source of information and strength rather than weakness.

It's not always easy to remember to practice noticing your feelings throughout the day. Perhaps wearing a rubber band that you can snap on your wrist will remind you to check inside to see how you are feeling, or you can set the alarm on your cell phone. You cannot learn about the thoughts and actions that cause your feelings until you are aware of your painful feelings. You cannot stop your addictive anesthetics until you are *willing* to feel your feelings and take responsibility for them.

If you decide you are willing to feel your feelings, that willingness will lead you to become more conscious of your feelings. This is the beginning of consciously choosing your intent to learn.

The willingness to take responsibility for your feelings also means you have the willingness to learn with your guidance so that you can access love and the wisdom to take loving action. You cannot fully feel your painful feelings and learn to take responsibility for them without a strong connection with your spiritual guidance.

I was motivated because I wanted to be able to make choices from love rather than from fear — choices that felt right inside and opened me to the richness of new possibilities. I let go of trying to have control over safety and became more of a risk taker. Trying to control feeling safe had done nothing but create anxiety for me.

Ironically, the more I practiced staying present for my feelings and connecting with my guidance, the safer I felt. And it wasn't until I had been practicing Inner Bonding for a few years that I felt true, deep joy for the first time in my life. Now I'm instantly aware the moment I feel something other than peace and fullness within. I quickly notice whether I've allowed my wounded self to think an untrue thought or something external is occurring that I need to attend to. I put my hand on my heart and compassionately embrace all feelings with the intention to learn, truly wanting responsibility for them, because I know from years of experience that this is the path to peace and joy.

Resistance Is Not More Important Than Loving Yourself

When my client Cecily was seven years old and her mother was beating her, she made a deep and profound decision: "I will not let her win. I will go inside and disconnect from myself so that she can't hurt me. She can beat me all she wants, but I will never show any emotion." Today, Cecily is forty-five years old and has spent her life disconnected from herself, operating from the false belief that this is the only way to not be hurt and controlled by anyone. She is miserable.

When my client Cameron was six years old and his father was beating him, he made the same decision: "I will not feel. I will not be present in my body, and then he cannot control me. I will win!" Cameron is in his early fifties. He is miserable.

Did you make a similar decision? Are you stuck in resisting to take responsibility for your feelings? Are you stuck in your unwillingness to feel your feelings and learn from them? Most people who have done even a little bit of Inner Bonding know the power it has to heal false beliefs and move them into truth. They know that they can develop their loving adult and discover the loving actions they can take for themselves. They know that they can learn to be loving advocates for themselves and to connect with their Divine guidance.

Why, then, do many people resist learning to love themselves? There are a number of reasons:

Some people resist because of a fear of ending up alone. Especially heterosexual woman can believe that they will become too healthy or too powerful and thus no men will be attracted to them. This is a huge false belief, because the healthier they get, the better chance they have of attracting other healthy people.

Some people believe that if they love themselves, they won't need anyone. But the truth is that the more we love ourselves, the more we want to learn and grow with others and share love with others. We will always need others for support — to have our backs — and we will always need others with whom to laugh, play, learn, grow, share affection, make love, and share love.

People might resist because of the fear of feeling the deep feelings of loneliness, heartbreak, and helplessness over others and events. Many people would unconsciously rather suffer from the stress of their wounded feelings than experience their existential painful feelings of life. Many people would rather be the cause of their own feelings — even when they don't want to acknowledge that they are causing them — because it makes them feel more in control. Many people want to avoid, at all costs, their existential painful feelings because feeling these feelings makes them feel out of control.

If you are unwilling to feel the painful feelings of life and learn how to manage them rather than avoid them, you will resist loving yourself, and you will continue to act out addictively. I have found that the feelings of loneliness and helplessness are very important feelings to experience. These feelings have much information for us.

Loneliness lets us know that someone is closed and emotionally unavailable and that we need to take care of ourselves in the face of that. Helplessness over others tells us when we need to let go of others and, again, take care of ourselves. When we open to these feelings and accept what they are telling us, we become empowered to take loving action for ourselves. If we fight these feelings, we never get the message they are trying to tell us, and we might keep hitting our heads against someone's wall or not taking the action we need for ourselves. To learn to love ourselves, we need to be willing to feel our deep, painful feelings.

Control and Resistance Might Be Your Gods

In his early sixties, my client Cole had been on a spiritual path for many years. He had attended meditation retreats, gone to years of therapy, and read all the latest self-help books. Still, he felt stuck. His marriage of five years was heading for divorce, and his business was getting nowhere. Cole was a deeply discouraged man when he first consulted with me.

Within the first couple of sessions, it became clear to me that all Cole's inner work had been coming from his wounded self. He was deeply intent on having control and not being controlled. His behavior in his relationship with his wife and with his employees was self-righteous, judgmental, and sometimes compliant on one hand and resistant on the other. He wanted control over how others felt about him while also having control over not being controlled by others.

Cole thought of himself as a kind, caring, and loving adult, yet all his behavior came from his wounded self with his desire to control and not be controlled. Unconsciously, control and resistance were his gods. Cole's intention to control caused his stuckness.

If you feel stuck in your life — if you feel frustrated, sad, alone, angry, depressed, and anxious — look at your intention. Chances are that control and resistance are your highest priorities rather than learning about loving yourself and others.

CHAPTER 14

INNER BONDING STEP 2: THE INTENT TO LEARN

The following is a comment from an InnerBonding.com online course member: "Listening to Dr. Margaret today, it finally made sense why for many years I longed for a higher-frequency spiritual connection but could not sustain it, as I was weighed down by negative thinking, severe hormonal problems, and food addiction. Now I am in menopause and eating clean foods, and it has become much easier to raise my vibration. My life has totally transformed. As my body has recovered, it has paved the way for the transformation of my thinking and taken me to a place where I am ready to transform my relationship with Spirit."

Our intention is crucial to our Divine connection. In every moment, each of us chooses our intention. For the most part, our intention originates from an attempt to control our lives, which to one degree or another can involve controlling our feelings or attempting to control others and the outcome of situations and events.

As I stated previously, we can simplify the choice of our intention by realizing that the intention we choose determines what actions we take and that there are only two choices in any given moment:

1. the intention to control in order to avoid pain
2. the intention to learn about loving ourselves and sharing our love with others

Step two of Inner Bonding is choosing the intention to learn:

Focus in your heart, consciously choosing the intention to learn to love yourself and others. Making this choice opens your heart, raises your frequency, and connects you with your compassionate Divine guidance, which is what creates your loving adult self.

Use any meditation or spiritual practice — or any other method — that helps you to surrender to your guidance and opens your heart to a compassionate intention to learn about how you are causing your wounded feelings and your false beliefs, how to lovingly manage your existential painful feelings, and what loving actions to take for yourself.

The Incredible Power of Intention

Intention is what governs how we think, feel, and behave. Our intent is the most powerful and creative force we have; it is the essence of free will. Our intent is our deepest desire, our primary motive or goal, our highest priority in any given moment.

Imagine two big spotlights. One is pointed upward, casting light far into the air. The other is pointed downward and buried in the earth; no light is cast at all. This is an example of intention.

When you consciously choose the intention to learn, your light points upward, shining on the truth that will guide you in your highest good. Your mind opens and becomes a receiver of the information you need to support yourself in manifesting your dreams. Consciously choosing the intention to learn about love is the most powerful thing we can do. Consciously choosing the intention to learn about loving ourselves is the second secret to connecting with our Divine guidance.

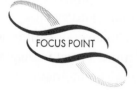
FOCUS POINT

Our intention governs us. It is the most powerful and creative force we have and the essence of free will.

When we unconsciously choose the intention to control, we shut off access to truth. Our minds become like closed-circuit TVs, recycling the old information that has been programmed into our egos. We become stuck in our limited wounded selves, operating from the false beliefs that we learned as we were growing up. We become stuck in the past, re-creating old hurts.

Our unconscious automatic choice is to control because of having to learn many ways to survive the pain of childhood. Most people immediately, and unconsciously, choose the intention to control the moment that they feel any anxiety or other pain. The problem is that the intention to control is self-abandoning, causing even more fear, anxiety, aloneness, emptiness, or depression. Instead of shining the light of love on your distress so that you learn and heal, you shove the light into the ground (like burying the spotlight in the earth), causing more darkness.

The challenge is to *remember* that we have a choice, to remember that we can choose the intention to learn about loving ourselves.

How can you remember to consciously choose the intention to learn? How can you remember in the moment you feel fear, anxiety, or stress to open to learning about what you are thinking or doing that is creating this stress? What can you do to stop your automatic reactive controlling and addictive behavior? How can you remember to open to learning rather than grab a donut? Practice!

You need to accept that choosing the intention to learn is an ongoing practice, not something that will occur quickly. We have all been practicing the intention to control for most of our lives, so it will take much practice to even remember that there is another choice.

Once you are aware of your painful feelings and you consciously want responsibility for them (step one), you can consciously choose to learn what you are thinking or doing that is causing your wounded feelings and what might be happening regarding a person or event that is causing your deeper painful feelings. Knowing this will enable you to make new choices to be more loving to yourself.

The intention to control disconnects you from your spiritual guidance, and the intention to learn connects you with your guidance. It's not always easy to discern your intention. The following checklists might help.

Checklist for Being Open to Learning

We are open to learning when we experience the following:

- We feel kindness and compassion — not judgment — for our feelings.
- We desire to take responsibility for our feelings and behavior.
- We know that we (and others) have good reasons for our feelings and behavior.
- We are genuinely curious about the good reasons for our feelings and behaviors — our fears and false beliefs.
- We are genuinely curious about our own and others' protective, controlling behaviors.
- We are connected with our Divine guidance.
- We are willing to tell our total truth without blame or judgment
- We are willing to risk losing others rather than lose ourselves.
- We know it is more important to be a loving human being than to protect against our fears of anger, judgment, rejection, failure, hurt, being controlled, and so on.
- We know it is more important to be a loving human being than attempt to have control over others making us feel temporarily safe, loved, happy, understood, adequate, successful, and so on.

Checklist for Being in the Intent to Control

We are protecting/avoiding/controlling when we choose the following thoughts and actions:

- We believe others are causing our wounded feelings of anger, anxiety, depression, guilt, shame, aloneness, and emptiness.
- We believe others are causing our behavior.
- We believe we are victims of others' choices.
- We believe we can control others' feelings or behaviors.
- We judge ourselves or others as right or wrong, good or bad
- We are unwilling to open to our Divine guidance.
- We are willing to lose ourselves rather than risk losing others.
- We are invested in outcomes because we attach happiness and a sense of worth to those outcomes and believe we can control them.
- We avoid taking responsibility for our feelings through protective, addictive, controlling behaviors.

Becoming aware of your intent moment by moment is one of the most important choices you can make. Health, vibrancy, Divine connection, freedom, and personal power come from being able to consciously choose the intention to learn about love rather than automatically and unconsciously having the intention to control. The more you become aware of your intent and consciously choose the intention to learn, the more you create the new neural pathways in your brain for being a loving adult.

It is of vital importance that you not judge yourself when you realize your intention is to control, because judging is just another way to control. Instead, choose to compassionately learn about your judgmental, controlling behavior. This is what leads to healing.

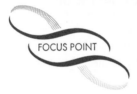

FOCUS POINT

The more you become aware of your intent and consciously choose the intention to learn, the more you create the new neural pathways in your brain for being a loving adult.

The Intention to Be Safe or Loving

Knowing our true intent is sometimes a tricky thing because sometimes intent is subtle, as my client Gordon discovered in one of my intensives. When he confessed he was feeling stuck, I asked him, "What do you think your intention is right now?"

"I came here to learn," he said without hesitation. "I'm very open to learning."

Although Gordon believed he was open to learning, in reality his ego was trying to be in control by appearing open to learning. Observing this, I invited him to tune in to what he was feeling right then and there.

"Anxious," he said, again without hesitation, giving the impression that he was very clear.

"Anxious," I echoed. "And what are you telling yourself that's causing you to feel anxious?"

Yet again, there wasn't a moment's hesitation. "That I have to get this."

"I see," I said, "so you're putting pressure on yourself to learn — which is to try to control the process of learning rather than actually being open to learning."

Gordon's eyes opened wide. "Oh my God, that's right!" he exclaimed. After a few moments to take in what was transpiring he added, "I think I do this all the time." The group was hushed. No one spoke as Gordon was evidently processing his discovery. A couple of minutes went by. When he again spoke, it was to announce to everyone, "Wow, I just experienced a huge sense of relief."

Confirming the difference in him, which was patently evident, I remarked, "That's because you actually opened up instead of your wounded self appearing to open."

True inner safety does not come from avoiding our fears. Avoidance only breeds more fear. True inner safety is the result of confronting our fears and developing a spiritually connected, loving adult to handle our fears of rejection, engulfment, loneliness, failure, and so on.

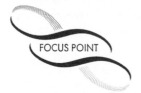

FOCUS POINT

True inner safety is the result of confronting fears and developing a spiritually connected loving adult to handle them.

The important thing here is not to rationalize, deny, and kid yourself into thinking that protecting yourself with your controlling and avoidant behavior is loving to yourself. Loving behavior is doing that which supports your highest good. Addictive, controlling, and avoidant behavior is never supportive of your highest good, even if it feels safe in the moment.

Be sure to ask yourself these questions in any given situation: "Is my intent really to be loving to myself, or am I just trying to be safe? Am I really focused on my highest good, or am I in denial in convincing myself that I'm being loving to myself?" Becoming aware of the intention to be safe from pain is what gives us the choice to learn to be loving to ourselves.

Divine Connection and the Intention to Learn

Since most of us did not have adequate role models for loving actions toward ourselves and others, our inner guidance can serve as our role model. It is, therefore, imperative to be able to easily and quickly connect with our inner guidance throughout the day.

Along with the vibrancy we attain from eating the way God intended us to eat, there is nothing else that I know of that raises our frequency high enough to access the love and wisdom of our Divine guidance than the intention to learn about love. But we can't fake this! We cannot act open and raise our frequency high enough to access our Divine guidance because acting open is just another form of control. Any attempt to control comes from the wounded self and will always lower our frequency. There is no way to access Divine guidance when our intention is to control, no matter how open we think we are. When the wounded self is in charge with the intent to control, our hearts are closed and our frequency is low.

From Wounded Self to Loving Adult

Once we are triggered into our wounded selves, it's often a challenge to get back to our openhearted loving adult. Remember, we are operating as a loving adult when our intention is to learn and we are connected with our Divine guidance.

Have you ever had the experience that you are going along fine, feeling peaceful inside, and then something happens that triggers you into your anxiety, anger, stress, hurt, fear, depression, and so on? Of course, it seems as if it is the external event that triggered you, such as someone yelling at you or blaming you; issues with money, children, or work; or rejection, engulfment, or other control issues. Now, instead of happily flowing along in your openhearted loving adult, your heart is closed, and you are stuck in your wounded self.

The stress in your body triggers thoughts that create even more stress, and you feel stuck in your anxiety or other painful feelings. How can you consciously move from your closed-hearted, controlling wounded self back into the open heart and intent to learn from your loving adult?

The most important choice you need to make after you are aware of your stressful feelings is that you really want to learn about what you are telling yourself, what you are believing, or what you are doing that is causing the stress. You can move into the intention to learn only from the place within you that wants responsibility for your feelings.

Along with choosing the intention to learn about loving yourself, there are some other choices you can make that will help you move into your spiritually connected, loving adult state. However, while all these choices can help you to raise your frequency, none will enable you to connect with your Divine guidance and become a loving adult unless you are also in the intention to learn.

Bridges to the Intention to Learn

When you are stuck in the anger, blame, depression, or numbness of your wounded self and you can't open to learning, you need to find a bridge that will take you into a state of openness to learning. Bridges are things you can do to open your heart.

The wounded self is always focused on the past and future, so one of the first things you can do is focus on this moment. If there is a lot of stress in your body, doing the emotional freedom technique (EFT) or the trauma release exercises (TRE) — you can learn both online — or doing some strenuous exercise such as running can move the stress out of your body and help you get present in the moment.

Of the many bridges you can use, prayer, especially a prayer of gratitude, is probably the most powerful. Prayer can take many forms, such as dialogue, meditation, chanting, recitation, or song. The choice is up to you. Some people have found that repeating a simple prayer of gratitude throughout the day helps them stay open to learning.

If you are too stuck in your woundedness to pray from your heart or you don't believe in prayer, then you need to try other bridges to open your heart to learn about love. Try one or more of the following:

- being in nature
- listening to heart-opening music
- deep breathing
- taking a walk
- gardening
- doing mundane activities, like the dishes or cleaning the house
- talking with a friend
- reading spiritual literature
- journaling
- smudging your environment with incense or with dried plants, such as sage, pine, cedar, or lavender

- drawing or doing other artwork, for example, sculpture or collage
- playing a musical instrument
- dancing
- attending twelve-step or other support group meetings
- playing with a child or a pet
- being held by a loving person
- letting yourself cry
- releasing your anger alone by yelling and pounding into a pillow (the Inner Bonding anger process[1])

Anger at another person is generally a projection of your inner child's anger at you for not taking loving care of yourself. Recognizing your anger at others as a projection can move you into the intent to learn.

In addition, open to your imagination. The willingness to move into and trust your imagination is very helpful in connecting with your Divine guidance. When you first begin to utilize your imagination, you might feel as if you are just making things up. However, as you take the risk of trusting what you think you are making up, you will discover that it is coming *through* you from your guidance rather than *from* you.

Of course, you also need to make sure you keep your body clear. As you already know, it is unlikely that you will be able to connect with your Divine guidance if you eat junk food or indulge in other substance addictions.

Notice Your Intent without Judgment

The heart of being in the intent to learn is to be willing to learn about our wounded, controlling behavior without judgment. It's when we are open to learning about our intent to control that we begin to have the consciousness and frequency we need to connect with our Divine guidance.

When we judge ourselves for our controlling, avoidant addictive behavior, we are trying to have control over getting ourselves

---

1. Learn about the Inner Bonding anger process here: http://www.innerbonding .com/show-article/296/managing-anger-the-inner-bonding-anger-process.html.

to change. We hope that by making ourselves wrong and "beating ourselves up," we will feel badly enough to change. But if you've ever really paid attention to the results of this, you might have noticed that the changes never occur. In fact, the more we judge ourselves and the worse we feel as a result of it, the more we want to act out with our addictions to avoid the pain of our self-judgments.

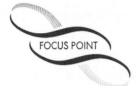

FOCUS POINT

When we are open to learning about our intent to control, we begin to have the consciousness and frequency we need to connect with our Divine guidance.

Giving up self-judgments is just as difficult as giving up any addictive behavior. The wounded self is deeply devoted to this form of control and doesn't want to let go of it. *So judging yourself for judging yourself will keep you stuck.*

You might want to think of being in the intent to learn about your intent to control as being on a treasure hunt. Uncovering the treasure of your false, limiting beliefs and the resulting controlling behavior is a great adventure, one that can lead to deep peace and joy.

Have Compassion for Your Wounded Self

Are you ignoring or judging your wounded self, hoping it will disappear? It is this very behavior that feeds the power and strength of your ego. Notice whether you are saying any of the following statements to yourself:

- "I hate my wounded self. I just want to get rid of her!"
- "My wounded self is ruining things for me. I wish he would just go away."
- "Maybe if I just ignore my wounded self, she will stop acting out."
- "Of course I judge my wounded self! How else can I get him to do things right?

Which part of you is saying these things? Your wounded self of course! And what happens when you judge or ignore your wounded self? It resists and acts out more. To have compassion rather than judgment for your ego, it's important to see who your wounded self really is:

- It's the scared part of you who had to learn — with your various addictions — how to control your feelings, others, and outcomes in order to survive. It's the part of you who had to ignore and repress your feelings to get through your childhood.
- It's the programmed part of you that absorbed — from your parents, teachers, friends, relatives, media, and religious training — lies about you, others, God, and what you can and cannot control. It's the part of you that feels separate from your Divine guidance and therefore feels alone.

It might help to see this part of you as a wounded child or adolescent who is doing the best he or she can to survive. You would not have gotten through your younger years with some sanity without your wounded self. Now, as an adult, this part is causing you problems because it is continuing to treat you the way you were treated or the way your parents treated themselves. Now, this part needs healing. But healing does not happen through judging or ignoring your ego.

You cannot heal your wounded self with your wounded self, and it is your wounded self who judges and ignores your feelings and behaviors and makes others responsible for you. You cannot heal inner abandonment with further inner abandonment. The only way to heal your wounded self is to fully embrace this part of you with a deep compassionate intention to learn.

The fears and beliefs of your wounded self that led to your addictive eating and other addictive behaviors will heal only through learning about them and bringing in the love and truth that you have always needed. You will continue to act from your wounded self as long as you feel unsafe. And the more you judge and ignore yourself and hand over to others the responsibility for your safety, the more unsafe you will feel.

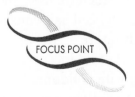

FOCUS POINT

You cannot heal your wounded self with your wounded self. You cannot heal inner abandonment with further inner abandonment.

We feel safe inside only when we feel seen, heard, and accepted with love and compassion. We do not feel safe when the only source of love and compassion is from another person. It is not safe to be dependent on a person because that person can always leave or die or be in a bad mood. You will feel safe only when there is a reliable source of love — which is you bringing love in from your Divine guidance. *Feeling safe is the result of letting go of junk foods and junk thoughts so that you have the vibrancy to connect with your Divine guidance.*

Your wounded self will not be willing to let go of junk food or junk thoughts until there is a strong, compassionate, spiritually connected loving adult willing to learn the truth and take the loving action necessary to create inner safety. Once there is a consistent, compassionate loving adult being guided by your Divine guidance and acting in your highest good, the wounded self will feel safe enough to release control.

Relationships are deeply affected when we are open to learning. Relationships flourish when both partners open to learning about themselves and each other. The best thing you can do to improve all your relationships is to focus on learning to love yourself so that you have love to share with your partner and others.

Intent is a simple concept but with such profound impact. Our society has been controlling to try to feel safe for a long time; clearly, it is not working. We will not feel safe until we do not feel alone within, and we will continue to feel alone within until we develop personal, ongoing spiritual connection so that we can operate as loving adults.

Our intent to protect automatically shuts out the very love and guidance we so desperately need. On the other hand, the moment we choose the intent to learn about loving, the heart opens and Divine love fills us. At that moment, with our Divine guidance surrounding us and filling us, we know that life is a privilege through which we are given the opportunity to heal and grow. Life never ceases to present us with challenges, but the intent with which we meet these challenges will determine whether life is experienced as a constant burden or a sacred privilege and a learning adventure.

Visualization Exercise for Connecting with Guidance

Sit somewhere that you are comfortable. You might want to play some soft music. It will be helpful to record this visualization exercise so that you can fully open to the experience of connecting with your Divine guidance.

Focus in your heart. Breathe into your heart, and consciously choose to be open to learning about loving yourself.

Imagine you are in a very beautiful place in nature. It can be the ocean, the mountains, a forest, or the desert. It can be a meadow. Perhaps there is a waterfall or a stream. Imagine that you can feel the temperature of the air on your skin; hear the sounds of the birds, the water, or the wind; smell the flowers, the trees, the salt, or the purity of the air; and even taste the air. Use all your senses as you imagine your beautiful place.

Imagine that you become aware of a warm, loving, powerful presence beside you. This presence is your Divine guidance. Your guidance wants to come in whatever form is comfortable for you, so you have an opportunity to imagine exactly how you want your guidance to appear to you. Depending on your worldview, picture a being or an energy, inside you or outside you, who for you is the most loving, powerful, and wise being or energy you could ever imagine. It could be a pure light or pure energy. It could be your experience of nature. It could be Jesus, Buddha, Krishna, Allah, Mother Mary, or one of the saints. It could be someone you have known and loved who has died. It could be the highest, most glorious part of you. Or it could be someone you make up — an inner mentor, a spirit guide, a guardian angel, or a teacher.

Your Divine guidance can be someone you see or something you feel — an energy of love, compassion, softness, power, strength, and wisdom. Just use your imagination and make up whatever feels completely safe, loving, wise, and powerful — a being or an energy or a light you would love to be held by or feel within you, a being or an energy or a light you can turn to for love and guidance. Imagine whatever feels most comfortable and safe for you.

Imagine that your Divine guidance is here now, and you feel surrounded by and filled with love. Imagine that you can relax and rest in the love of your Divine guidance. If this is a being other than your higher self or someone you know, you can make up whatever name you like for this being.

Imagine the peace that surrounds you and is within you as

you are with this energy of love. Imagine that your guidance knows everything about you and loves you unconditionally. Imagine that your guidance never leaves you and is always with and within you. This is your personal source of Divine guidance, and you can always turn to it for love, wisdom, strength, and truth.

Once you open to your guidance, invite in the loving, compassionate presence of Spirit by simply saying, "I invite you into my heart. I invite compassion and wisdom into my heart."

Now you are in the loving adult state, and you are ready for step three of Inner Bonding.

CHAPTER 15

INNER BONDING STEP 3: DIALOGUE WITH THE WOUNDED AND CORE SELVES

Once you are focused in your heart and feel kind and open to your feelings, then you can move into step 3 of the Inner Bonding process:

Compassionately dialogue with your inner child to discover your thoughts and false beliefs and the resulting behaviors that cause the painful wounded feelings you tuned in to in step 1. Open to exploring what happened as you were growing up that created your loneliness, heartbreak, and helplessness concerning others and the resulting false beliefs that have led to your self-abandonment. Compassionately embrace your existential painful feelings. Explore your gifts and what brings joy to your core self.

In step 3, you will open your heart to all aspects of yourself — your wounded aspects as well as your core, feeling self. Look at this as an exploration into the layers of you. When you talk to your angry, hurt, frightened, anxious, numb, guilty, shamed, needy, or depressed inner child, welcome and embrace those feelings, whatever they are. Your job is to welcome him or her into your loving embrace so that you can learn what you are believing, thinking, or

doing that causes these painful feelings. Ask your inner child —
your core self — these questions:

- "What am I telling you or doing that makes you feel anxious (or
  depressed, angry, shamed, and so on)?"
- "Are you angry with me? It's okay to be angry with me."
- "Am I letting you down or not taking care of you in some way?
  How?"
- "How do you feel when I give you junk food — or drugs or alco-
  hol — or avoid you with any other addiction when you are feeling
  lonely, hurt, bored, anxious, depressed, or angry?"
- "What do you really want from me when you feel bad?"
- "What do you need from me right now?"
- "How am I abandoning you? Am I making others responsible for
  you? Am I judging you? Am I ignoring your feelings and needs and
  not listening to you? Am I discounting you? Am I numbing you
  with substances or activities?"

None of these statements are written in stone; feel free to draft
your own. It is very important for you to tune in to what your unique
essence needs to hear from you and the kinds of questions that help
your soul open to you.

No feelings are ever wrong or bad. All the painful, wounded feelings you have are for good reasons — these are your fears and false
beliefs — and by gently using step 3's dialogue process with great
kindness and compassion, you will be able to discover the information these feelings are trying to tell you.

You will explore — with love, gentleness, compassion, and curiosity — not only your feelings but also whatever related false beliefs,
behaviors, and memories you might have. For some people, using a
doll or stuffed animal to represent their core selves is very helpful.
You can hold this surrogate child and bring yourself comfort when
painful feelings come up. It is best to dialogue out loud or in writing.
Both speaking out loud and writing slows the process down so that
you can hear it.

Once you understand what you are telling yourself and how you
are treating yourself, you can then dialogue with various aspects
and ages of your wounded self. You dialogue with your wounded self

about the false beliefs that are causing your self-abandoning behavior, which is causing your painful, wounded feelings.

The following is a very brief example of a dialogue. In this example, a woman in one of my intensives decided to work with me, and she felt very anxious.

⤸

Adult: What am I telling you or doing that is making you feel anxious?

Child: You are telling me that I have to do this right, and I don't know how. You are telling me that if I don't do it right, others will judge me and I will be rejected.

Adult: Yes, I have been telling you that. How do you feel when I tell you this?

Child: I feel like you won't like me unless I do everything right and prove that I am worthy. I always feel I have to prove that I'm okay to you and everyone else. You keep telling me not to make a fool of myself.

Adult: So of course you feel anxious. Wow! I tell myself these things a lot, and I always thought my anxiety was coming from other people. I'm the one who is causing it!

[The woman then spoke with the wounded self.]

Adult: There must be a good reason you keep telling the inner child she has to do everything right. What are you trying to control or avoid feeling by focusing on doing everything right?

Wounded self: I want people to like me.

Adult: So you believe that you can have control over how people feel about you by doing things right?

Wounded self: Yes.

⤸

After such a dialogue, you would go to step 4, which is in the next chapter, and ask your Divine guidance what is true and what is loving to you.

You can dialogue with your core self when you experience life's painful feelings, compassionately keeping yourself company when you feel loneliness, grief, sorrow, heartache, heartbreak, and help-lessness concerning others and events. You can also dialogue with your core self about what you love to do, exploring your gifts, pas-sions, and talents; what brings you joy; what is your true calling; and what fulfills your soul.

Suggestions for Successful Dialoguing

A very important aspect of dialoguing is to be aware of who is ask-ing the questions: Is it your loving adult or your wounded self? At any given moment, we are either operating as loving adults or our pro-grammed wounded selves.

Are you really in a compassionate intent to learn (as your loving adult), or are you asking the questions from your fear and pain (as your wounded self)? Do you want to learn about how you might be causing your pain (your loving adult), or are you just trying to get rid of the pain (your wounded self)? You will not receive helpful or accu-rate answers when your wounded self asks the questions. This is why it is imperative to do steps 1 and 2 before starting to dialogue.

Listen to the Answers

When you are ready to hear the answer to your questions, move your attention into your body. The answers will come from deep within you rather than from your mind.

You will find you gradually let go of your addictions when you attend to your feelings whenever you feel anything other than peace and fullness inside. Instead of turning to junk food or another form of self-abandonment, you will find out what you really want by dia-loguing with your core self. You might ask, "What is it you are *really* seeking or feeling hungry for?" The wounded self always grabs for a short-term fix — your favorite junk food, new clothes, sex, TV, alco-hol, pot, or cocaine are some examples. But by embracing and listen-ing to your feelings, you can discover what you really want and need.

Of course, the answer is always love and connection, as well as any number of loving actions. Your inner self wants to experience Divine love coming through your loving adult from your Divine guidance. It is only when you learn to bring through divine, unconditional love to yourself that the hunger, emptiness, and aloneness you experience are relieved. Until you address the issue of your inner aloneness and emptiness — the aloneness and emptiness that you have been filling with your junk food and various other addictions — you cannot begin to address the issue of the loneliness you might feel with others or from not having others around, as well as past and present heartache, heartbreak, grief, and helplessness concerning others and events.

You will feel both alone and lonely until you heal your aloneness, your separation from Divine love. By opening to learning with your feelings, you can discover the fears and false beliefs that are in the way of your receiving Divine love.

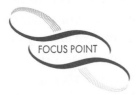

FOCUS POINT

When you learn to bring through divine, unconditional love to yourself, the hunger, emptiness, and aloneness you experience are relieved.

Clarify the Dialogue Process

The most important aspect of dialoguing is to make sure that you are in your loving adult self and are open to learning and experiencing compassion for your feelings. If you sense any wounded feelings, then ask, "What am I telling you and how am I treating you to cause these feelings?" Your inner child might say something similar to the following:

- "You are telling me I'm not good enough."
- "You are ignoring me."
- "You are stuffing me down with food."
- "You keep giving me away to others for approval."

The part of you who is abandoning your inner child with judgments by staying in your head or through various addictions is your ego. Ask your wounded self, "What are you trying to control or avoid feeling by judging" (or by overeating or eating junk food, staying in your head, or making others responsible for you) "the inner child?" This is where you begin to discover your false beliefs.

Your wounded self might be able to tell you what he or she is trying to control or avoid feeling with the self-abandoning behavior. Once you get a clear picture of how you are treating yourself and the beliefs behind your unloving behavior toward yourself, then you can move to step 4 and ask, "What is the truth about these false beliefs?" and "What is the loving action needed toward my inner child?" (We will get to this in the next chapter.)

When you tune in to your feelings (**step 1**) and discover core painful feelings (such as loneliness, heartache or heartbreak, or helplessness concerning others) and you are certain that you are open to compassionate learning (**step 2**), then hold your inner child with love and kindness, letting him or her know that you are not alone (**step 3**). Putting your hands on your heart helps with this. You need to let your core self know that you understand why he or she is feeling this way in the particular situation, event, or interaction. Your inner child needs to feel seen, loved, and understood. Once you feel calm, you can ask your guidance, "What is important for me to learn in this situation?" and "What is the loving action I need to take?" (**step 4**).

With practice, this will become clearer. With wounded feelings, you always want to discover the false beliefs that fuel your self-abandoning behavior, and then you want to start to heal these false beliefs by turning to your Divine guidance for the truth and taking loving action for yourself (**step 5**) based on the truth. This is what gradually heals your false beliefs.

Lies from the Wounded Self

Our wounded selves are constantly telling us lies about ourselves and about how things are in order to have control over getting us to do things "right." A major part of the exploration process is discovering the lies we tell ourselves that are causing our pain. While truth comes from our Divine guidance, the lies we tell ourselves come from our programmed ego, our wounded minds. Our wounded selves are masters at judging us and creating lies.

The wounded self has hundreds of beliefs about us, control, others, and God that cause us much pain. When we believe these lies, we end up feeling depressed, anxious, empty, angry, guilty, shamed, hurt, or scared. When we feel these feelings, it is generally because we believe a lie that our wounded selves have told us (other than the anxiety and depression caused by a toxic gut). These feelings are our inner guidance's way of telling us that we are abandoning and lying to ourselves.

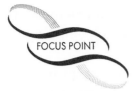

FOCUS POINT

Discover the lies you are telling yourself that cause your pain. These come from your wounded self.

To disempower the lies and judgments of the wounded self, you need to do the following:

1. Become aware of what you are telling yourself by staying tuned in to your feelings in step 1 and noticing when you are feeling bad and then moving to step 2 — the intent to learn. Ask yourself, "What am I telling myself that is making me feel bad?"

2. Next, ask yourself, "Am I 100 percent certain that what I am telling myself is true?" The chances are you will recognize that you have made up the lie that is causing your pain.

3. Then ask the question (step 4), "What is the truth?" When you have a sincere desire to know the truth and your vibrancy is high enough from clean eating, the answer will come to you from your Divine guidance.

4. Consciously bring the truth to the wounded part of you, and take action based on that truth. Over time, your inner dialogue will shift from lies to truth. Truth frees you from the lies and from the painful feelings that result from the lies.

   - Instead of, "She doesn't like me because I'm not smart enough," the inner statement might be, "She looks like she's having a hard time today."
   - Instead of, "I can't do it right. Now I'm in trouble," the statement might be, "There might be something interesting to learn with this person."
   - Instead of, "I'll never get this right. I'll never be okay," the statement might be, "This is an interesting challenge. I'm going to keep at this until I really understand it."
   - Instead of, "I'm such a jerk. How could I have said such a thing?" the statement might be, "I wonder why I said that? There must be a good reason."
   - Instead of, "Life is a losing battle. I'll never get anywhere," the statement might be, "Life is a sacred privilege of learning about love, and I'm going to keep on learning!"

- Instead of, "It's always my fault," the statement might be, "There must be a good reason this is happening. I wonder what my part is?"
- Instead of, "I'll always be alone," the statement might be, "I can't predict the future, but I'm actually never alone. My Divine guidance is always here with me."

Manage Life's Painful Feelings

My experience from years of counseling people individually and as couples is that most of the problems people suffer from stem from how they handle the life events rather than the events themselves. Certainly traumatic and tragic events (loss of loved ones, financial loss, war, rape, and health issues) are extremely challenging. However, some people manage to move through these events with equanimity while others remain stuck in fear, anxiety, anger, and depression. The difference is in how people handle deep painful feelings and traumatic events.

Loneliness is an intensely sad, sinking, or burning feeling within. This feeling can be triggered from numerous situations, such as the following:

- loss of a loved one
- not having a partner, family, or friends with whom to share time and love
- being around others but being closed off to them
- being around others when they are closed off to you

Other than a traumatic loss, the latter is often the most challenging in everyday life, and this can occur throughout the day. For example, you walk into work happy and open. You greet your coworker, and he or she barely responds to you. If you are truly open to your feelings, you will feel a stab of loneliness. However, most people are so closed off to this feeling that they immediately attempt to avoid the feeling with some kind of addictive behavior. They might grab a doughnut while shaming or blaming — telling themselves that they must have done something wrong or that the coworker is being a jerk.

These addictive behaviors work for the moment to appease the feeling, but the feeling doesn't actually go away. It just goes deeper within and could eventually cause physical symptoms, such as back pain or some form of illness.

Heartbreak can occur in many different situations. Here are a few examples:

- loss — of a loved one, health, or financial security
- people being unloving toward you, others, animals, or the planet
- people harming themselves

Helplessness is a feeling of intense inner turmoil. In the example of greeting your coworker and receiving a cold response, not only do you have the stab of loneliness but you also feel the pain of helplessness over your coworker's behavior. You cannot make him or her connect with you. However, because this is such a difficult feeling, you don't want to know that you cannot have control over another or over the outcome of things. To avoid knowing about your lack of control, you might shame yourself: "It's my fault. If I'm different, I can get others to be different." Or you might blame your coworker, attempting to get him or her to change. Both shame and blame are attempts to avoid accepting helplessness concerning others and events.

Once you turn to addictive behaviors, you have abandoned yourself. In attempting to avoid feeling the loneliness, heartbreak, and helplessness, you have created inner aloneness through your self-abandonment. The combination of avoiding loneliness, heartbreak, helplessness, and the aloneness that comes from inner abandonment can lead to anxiety, depression, and despair. People often turn to prescription drugs to further avoid their feelings.

Managing the feelings of loneliness, heartbreak, and helplessness is not as hard as you might think. If you practice the following aspects of Inner Bonding, you will find that you do not need to use your various addictions to avoid pain.

Stay tuned in to your body/feelings (step 1) so that you know when you are feeling lonely, heartbroken, helpless concerning others, sorrow, grief, shattered, or crushed. It's helpful to be able to acknowledge and name the feeling, and it might take some time to recognize these feelings since you might have been avoiding them for a long time. Consciously decide that you want responsibility for nurturing and then releasing these feelings.

Welcome and embrace the feelings; open to them with deep compassion. Connect with your spiritual source of love and compassion. Open to this Source, and ask for help in being kind and compassionate toward these feelings.

Hold the feelings as you would a child who is hurting — with deep love and understanding. Just be with the feelings, accepting them, for a few minutes.

Open to learn about what the feelings are telling you about a person or a situation and about what would be the loving action toward the person or situation.

Dialogue with the feelings to gain the understanding you need about the person or situation.

Consciously be willing to release the feelings. Imagine the painful feelings moving through you and being released into the universe — into Divine love. Ask Spirit to replace these feelings with acceptance and inner peace.

You will find that these painful feelings will release if you practice these steps rather than abandon yourself in the face of painful events and experiences. With huge losses, you will need to do this every time the pain comes up, and you might need to ask others for help and comfort.

Relationships Can Trigger Deeper Pain

"I work hard to get into a centered and connected place," my client Jenna shared with me. "I'll be doing great when, out of nowhere, Seth blames me for something, and it all goes out the window. I get upset with him for blaming me when I'm trying my best. It makes me feel off-center and down for days." Jenna fell silent for a few moments. Then she suggested, "Maybe I shouldn't be with him? Maybe my inner guidance is telling me I'd be better off without him so that I can stay in a good space?"

I didn't hesitate to clarify what was really happening. "While it's hard for you to see this right now, Seth is providing you with a wonderful opportunity to learn to stay centered and connected even in the face of his wounded ego. Can you imagine being able to do this? Can you imagine how good it would feel to stay connected with yourself even when he is disconnected?"

"Is that what I'm doing, disconnecting from myself?" Jenna asked, looking puzzled.

"Any time we're angry, upset, blaming, or distant, we've disconnected from ourselves. You're being triggered into coming from your wounded self as a result of Seth being in his wounded self."

Still looking puzzled, Jenna pressed, "But how do I not do that? I feel so upset when Seth doesn't appreciate my efforts. Shouldn't I let him know how I feel? Am I supposed to just be nice and hold my feelings in?"

"Your upset feelings are important, and you don't want to ignore them," I confirmed. "But when you get angry at Seth, you are ignoring your feelings. Take a moment right now to see what the deeper feelings are when Seth blames you. What's going on inside you?"

Tearing up, Jenna said, "My mother constantly blamed me for her feelings. Everything was my fault."

"How did that feel to you as a child?"

"It felt like I couldn't do anything right."

"Precisely. So what I want you to do now is breathe into that feeling. There's a deeper feeling beneath it. When you access it, tell me what you experienced when you felt you couldn't do anything right."

After several moments, Jenna responded, "I felt crushed, so crushed."

"Is that how you feel when Seth blames you instead of appreciates you?"

"It's exactly how I feel."

"Jenna, if you had a little girl who was feeling crushed, what would she need from you?"

Jenna thought for a minute. Then she said, "She would need for me to hold her and understand her feelings."

"Yes, and this is exactly what you need to do for your inner child when Seth blames you. Instead, you abandon yourself, completely disconnecting in order to retaliate against Seth. This is why you end up feeling so bad. The next time Seth blames you, I hope you'll be willing to try something different. The moment he blames you, put your hands on your heart and breathe into your heart, connecting with the compassion of your spiritual center. Then bring that compassion to the crushed feeling you are experiencing. Hold the feeling with compassion and tenderness until it begins to dissipate. Are you willing to try this?"

After a few weeks of practice, Jenna reported that she was thrilled with being able to stay centered and connected whenever Seth blamed her for something or showed a lack of gratitude. She found that instead of lashing out to try to control him, if she just went inside, she soon felt good again. To her surprise, Seth also seemed to be blaming her less and less.

Following is a dialogue example to use when you become aware of feeling anxious (or some other wounded feeling).

- In **step 1**, breathe into the anxiety, moving toward the feeling, embracing it with kindness, sitting with it, and being fully present with the feeling of anxiety. Find a place in your heart that wants responsibility for how you are treating yourself or what you are telling yourself that is causing this feeling.

- In **step 2**, focus on your heart. Breathe in and out, getting fully present in your heart. Consciously choose to learn about how you are treating yourself and the false beliefs behind your self-abandoning behavior. Invite love and compassion into your heart by simply saying to your Divine guidance, "I invite your love and compassion into my heart." You are in a loving adult state when you are compassionately intent on learning to love yourself and you feel connected with your Divine guidance.

- In **step 3**, ask the anxious part of you (your inner child), "What am I telling you or how am I treating you that is making you feel anxious?"

Child: You are telling me that I have to know what I'm doing and not make any mistakes. I have to do everything right, and if I don't, then I'm not good enough.

Adult: Yes, that's what I'm telling you. I see I'm putting a lot of pressure on you, and that makes you anxious.

Now the loving adult turns to the wounded self to discover the false belief:

Adult: There must be a good reason we are putting so much pressure on the child and telling the child that we can't make a mistake.

How old were we when we started to put this pressure on ourselves? (At any given moment, the wounded self can be any age from prebirth up through our twenties, depending when we absorbed a particular belief.)

Wounded self: I think this started when we were about seven. That's when Mom and Dad started to get angry when I didn't make straight As.

Adult: So you believe that being perfect and not making mistakes is the way to get love?

Wounded self: Yes. That's the only way we got any attention and when they weren't angry with us.

Adult: So now you believe that you can control how others feel about us by being perfect?

Wounded self: Yes. We have to get love to be okay. If someone judges us, then it proves that we are not good enough.

Adult: So you believe that our worth is determined by others' approval?

Wounded self: Yes! Of course!

Adult: What do you think would happen if we didn't pressure and judge ourselves?

Wounded self: I think we would sit around and do nothing. The only way we are motivated to do well is to be hard on ourselves, put pressure on ourselves, and judge ourselves.

At this point, you would go to step 4 and dialogue with your Divine guidance about the truth of all the false beliefs you uncovered. You would ask for the truth about the following false beliefs:

- "Can I have control over getting love by being perfect?"
- "Is my worth determined by how others feel about me?"
- "If we didn't judge and pressure ourselves, would we sit around and do nothing?"
- "Do we motivate ourselves by being hard on ourselves?"

We will answer these questions in the next chapter.

CHAPTER 16

INNER BONDING STEP 4: DIALOGUE WITH YOUR HIGHER GUIDANCE

Once you understand which of your thoughts, false beliefs, and actions are causing you pain, you are ready to learn the truth about those beliefs and discover what new, loving action you need to take for yourself. This information will come to you through a dialogue with your Divine guidance — step 4.

The Challenge of Divine Connection

In her book, *My Stroke of Insight*, brain scientist Jill Bolte Taylor, PhD, describes her devastating stroke at the age of thirty-seven from a congenital deformation of a blood vessel in her brain. Her entire left brain was flooded with blood, rendering her unable to move, talk, or think in the usual way. Because her left brain went offline, her right brain was free to take over, and she had a profound experience of inner peace, joy, and sense of oneness with the universe. Dr. Taylor was stunned to discover that her soul was huge and fluid and able to freely move around the universe. She was also stunned to discover that she was actually a temporary visitor in her body and that she was not her body.

With great effort and the loving help of her mother and others, she was eventually able to heal her left brain. In the process, she decided that she no longer wanted the angry, defensive, controlling parts of her programmed left brain (her ego) to be in charge, and she learned many ways to allow her right brain to be in charge. Because she had such a profound experience of spiritual connection when her left brain was not functioning, she has moved into deep faith and Divine connection in her life.

While Dr. Taylor eventually received great gifts from the stroke, this is a very traumatic way of moving into connection and faith! The rest of us can connect without having our left brains go offline. Interestingly, when she could no longer access her left-brain mind, she could still think. She (her higher self) was able to observe what was going on the whole time. Being a brain scientist at Harvard, Dr. Taylor was extremely interested in what was going on in her brain.

The wounded self is always worried that we will "lose our minds" if we let go of control, but nothing of the sort happened to Dr. Taylor. In fact, she was able to be in her "right mind" the whole time. Suddenly, she was able to relate to people, not from their outer form as she previously had, but from their energy. She instantly knew when someone was controlling, needy, and taking energy from her, as well as when someone was loving, caring, and giving energy to her. She had so little energy after her stroke that she would leave her body and fly around the universe when a controlling, needy person was with her!

What all this says to me is part of the challenge of being divinely connected is disciplining ourselves to not indulge our wounded selves with those programmed judgmental thoughts and instead to "step to the right" and "tend the garden of our minds,"[1] as Dr. Taylor puts it. In reading her book, I was very impressed with how vigilant she is in not allowing her wounded self to take over. After experiencing such incredible peace and joy, she is deeply motivated to experience peace and joy as often as she can.

---

1. Jill Bolte Taylor, PhD, *My Stroke of Insight* (London: Penguin Books, 2009) pp. 176–177.

Connecting with Spirit Is Simple But Not Always Easy

- "I keep asking Spirit questions, but I just don't hear anything."
- "I'm trying every day to connect with my guidance, but nothing is happening."
- "I think I just don't have a knack for this spiritual connection thing."
- "Aren't I supposed to hear something?"
- "Is it supposed to be this hard?"

Actually, it's not hard at all. We all have the built-in wiring to connect with Spirit. It's our birthright to have this connection, just as it is a baby's birthright to have a parent's connection and guidance.

When your frequency is high because you have a pure intent to learn about what is loving to you and because you are eating clean, guidance will be right there. However, as I've previously stated, the wounded self is very tricky. It can trick us into thinking we are open to learning when, in fact, it has a very different intention — to control something. Do you want to know what is loving to you because you want to be loving or so that you can get rid of pain? Do you want to learn in order to get something — love, approval, money, a new job, or a partner — or because you truly want to evolve your ability to love yourself and others?

While you might consciously think your intention is to love yourself and support your highest good, your unconscious intention in that moment might be very different, and it is this deeper intention that governs whether or not you connect with your guidance. The wounded self always has an agenda in mind and thinks it can trick Spirit into giving you guidance for that agenda by acting open. But Spirit can't be tricked or fooled.

The problem is that our guidance can't communicate with us unless we are truly open. When the wounded self is in charge, our frequency is not high enough for us to access Spirit or for Spirit to access us. There is no opening through which Spirit can communicate with us unless we have a true intention to learn about loving ourselves and our vibrancy is high from eating well.

When your deepest desire is to control rather than learn about loving yourself and others — and your intention is to get rid of your feelings rather than learn from them — you will not be able to access your Divine guidance even if you are eating a perfect diet. Connecting with your guidance is easy when your deepest desire is to evolve into a more loving human being — with yourself and with others. When you have the courage to take loving action for yourself (such as standing up for yourself, telling your truth, taking risks to discover your joy, taking care of yourself physically through diet and exercise, or feeling your painful feelings and learning about what you might be doing to create your pain), then your Divine guidance will show you the way. Your guidance will find a way to communicate with you when your vibrancy is high from a clean nutrient-dense diet and your pure desire is to learn about love, starting with loving yourself.

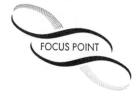

FOCUS POINT

When your deepest desire is to control rather than learn about loving yourself and others, you will not be able to access your Divine guidance, even if you are eating a perfect diet.

When you are ready to learn how to take loving care of yourself, then ask your Divine guidance how to do it, and you will be shown the way. Your guidance is just waiting for you to ask.

Spirit's job is to guide us in our highest good. Our guidance is always hanging around, just waiting for the opportunity to help us. But because we have free will, Spirit cannot do anything about our intent or our frequency. We are 100 percent in charge of our intention to love or our intention to control and whether we choose to eat in a way that fosters Divine connection.

When you practice dialoguing with your Divine guidance, asking questions and "imagining" the answers, eventually you will feel and know through your experiences that Spirit is actually helping and guiding you. You will develop a relationship with your Divine guidance. You will find that answers to your questions come more easily, and you will know from personal experience that you are never alone. When you imagine your guidance (in any form) with an intention to learn about becoming a more loving human being and you have raised your vibrancy with your diet, you can access the comfort, power, love, compassion, peace, joy, and wisdom that is available to you.

Imagining a being of light — or light itself — surrounding you with love can energize your being and bring you great comfort. Being connected with Spirit is like being connected with an infinite source of power. It is the difference between trying to light your way with a small flashlight powered by rundown batteries or with a huge lamp plugged into an industrial-strength wall socket. Our wounded selves are exhausted from running on batteries. All we need to do is plug into the infinite Source available to us to energize our beings.

How Spirit Guides You

As I've previously stated, one way our guidance is always communicating with us is through our emotional feelings. Our emotions are an inner guidance system, instantly letting us know whether we are thinking and behaving in ways that are on or off track regarding our highest good. This is why it is so important to be aware of your feelings.

Sometimes you might hear an actual voice, or ideas could pop into your mind. Whole concepts might suddenly occur to you. You might receive pictures of loving actions, or your dreams might be a powerful source of guidance. You might read it in a book that someone happened to send you, hear it from your voice as you're helping someone, or hear it from someone else. It might come in meditation or when you are in the shower. However it comes, it will come when your intention is pure. Whatever form your answers come in, know that they will light the way for your next step.

You will know that you are receiving actual guidance by how you feel. The truth and the loving action from your guidance make you feel peaceful, and the lies and false beliefs from your wounded self make you feel distressed.

The universe is filled with the energy of love and truth. It is filled with all the information there is, and it has the answers to all our questions. Asking your guidance questions about the truth of your beliefs and about what loving behavior you can take for yourself will eventually result in answers, but sometimes they do not come immediately. They might pop into your mind when you least expect it.

When you sincerely ask the questions, "What is the truth about this belief?" and "What is the loving action in this situation?" you open the channel for this information to come through you. We have long been told to "ask and you shall receive." Try it. It really works.

What Your Guidance Tells You

My experience with my guidance is that she never imposes anything on me. She answers my questions in a way that makes me feel calm and peaceful rather than scared. She never tests me, and she would never tell me disturbing things or try to jolt me into action. She is unconditionally kind, caring, comforting, supportive, wise, compassionate, loving, and powerful. I would not know how to live my life without her.

My clients often ask me: "I attempt to communicate with my higher guidance every day, but how can I be sure that what is being relayed to me isn't just my ego? How do I know the difference between the lies coming from my wounded self and the truth coming from Spirit? When I think I am receiving information from Spirit, how do I know that I'm not just making it up?"

Knowing the difference between Spirit's truth and the lies of the wounded self is a learning process, a process of discernment. Discernment comes when we are present with our feelings. If your heart is heavy and constricted and you are unaware of it, you will not get the message that your heart is trying to give you. Truth opens the heart. Lies close it. Your feelings are meant to guide you, to let you know when you are operating from truth and when you are stuck in lies. The feelings of the gut and the heart are very accurate guides.

When we tune out our feelings with our addictions, we have no way of knowing the difference between lies and truth — between the beliefs that come from our limited ego minds and the truth that comes directly from Spirit. When we immediately go to food, drugs, alcohol, busyness, TV, anger, withdrawal, compliance, resistance, or any other addictive process, we effectively close our hearts and cut off our feelings, which cuts off our discernment of lies and truth.

We have been blessed with a fail-safe system of knowing what is right and true for us. When I receive a thought or image, I check in with my feelings to see whether it feels right inside. When it feels right, I know it is from my Divine guidance. If something about it doesn't feel right, then I'm suspicious that it is coming from my wounded self. I stay open and ask my guidance for clarity. When the thoughts and images I receive line up with what feels right inside, I know I am on the right track.

When we feel peaceful and full of love, we know that we are taking loving care of ourselves. When we feel anxious, depressed, angry, ashamed, or jealous, we know we are abandoning ourselves. Our Divine guidance is here to guide us in what is loving for us. Our guidance tells us what is true and what is loving for ourselves and others.

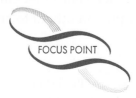

Our guidance is here to guide us in what is true and loving to ourselves and others.

Ask the Right Questions

If you want your guidance to give you answers that will help you, then you need to ask the right questions. The right questions always have to do with truth and loving action for yourself.

The right questions are not about the future and the outcome of things. These questions are from the wounded self and are about control, and this is not what your guidance supports you in. Your guidance is here to love and comfort you; guide you in your highest good; bring love, peace, joy, and compassion into your heart; and teach you the truth about your false beliefs. The right questions are like these:

- "What is the truth about this belief that I have uncovered in step 3 of Inner Bonding?"
- "What is the loving action I need to take for my inner child?
- "What is in my highest good right now?"
- "What does my inner child need from me right now to feel safe inside?"
- "What does my inner child need from me right now to feel safe in this conflict with _____?"
- "What does my inner child need from me right now to feel loved by me?"
- "What do I need to do differently for my inner child to feel safe in an interaction with _____?"

When you ask these questions about love and truth with a deep and sincere desire to learn, you put out into the universe that you really want to know how to take responsibility for your feelings and well-being. This is what Divine guidance responds to.

Notice that these questions are all about the truth and loving action toward you — not about loving others or what is the truth for them. Trying to be loving to others without first being loving to yourself is about control, and your guidance will not answer these questions. When you are loving to yourself, you will naturally be loving to others, but if you try to be loving to others first, then your inner child will feel abandoned, and you will energetically pull on others to give you the love that you are not giving yourself.

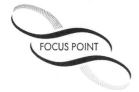

FOCUS POINT

Trying to be loving to others without first being loving to yourself is about control, and your guidance will not answer these questions.

Receive the Truth from Your Guidance

At the end of the last chapter, there were a number of beliefs uncovered in a dialogue using step 3:

- "Can I have control over getting love by being perfect?"
- "Is my worth determined by how others feel about me?"
- "If we didn't judge and pressure ourselves, would we sit around and do nothing?"
- "Do we motivate ourselves by being hard on ourselves?"

When I started practicing Inner Bonding and I asked my guidance about the truth of these same beliefs, here is what she said:

> Love is always a gift and not subject to control. Sometimes you can control getting approval but never love, and it's important not to confuse love with approval.
>
> You are already perfect in your essence. Your wounded self wants to believe that there is some standard of perfection that you can live up to and that will earn you love, but love can't be earned, and there isn't some standard to live up

to. Since your essence is a perfect individual expression of God, your worth is intrinsic. The more you open to knowing who you uniquely are, the more you will value yourself. Eventually, you won't even think about how others feel about you.

When you judge and put pressure on yourself, you make it harder to do what you want to do. There is often a tendency to resist the inner control. Contrary to sitting around and doing nothing, loving yourself will energize you to take loving action. Your essence is intrinsically motivated and doesn't need judgment and pressure to pursue that which expresses who you are.

Trust Your Inner Guidance

You might find it challenging to trust your guidance. I often hear my clients say, "I hear my guidance, but I don't believe it is my guidance," or "I hear my guidance, but I don't trust that what I'm hearing is true or right."

I understand this issue well, as it took me years after starting to practice Inner Bonding to trust my guidance more than my wounded self. I needed to test it. How could I be sure that what was coming *through* my mind was truer than what came *from* my mind? How could I be sure it really was Spirit? I tested and tested. I noticed what happened when I didn't listen and what happened when I did. Finally, I was able to fully accept that my guidance is here for me and that she knows what is good and right for me. I fully accepted that my wounded self is a programmed survival part of me that has no access to truth or love.

Now when I have a thought that creates anxiety, I immediately dismiss the thought as being made up by my wounded self. I know that my guidance never gives me thoughts that create anxiety. I also know that definitive thoughts about the future — about what will or won't happen — are generally made-up thoughts from my wounded self. The wounded self loves to predict the future, and the loving adult stays in the present, connected with the truth of the moment.

However, my guidance often tells me what to do in the present that will greatly affect the future, such as when she loudly told me to slow down on the freeway so that the drunk driver wouldn't hit me or when she told me to get everything of value out of my house a week before my house closed escrow in 2001 — a week before I was supposed to move. I didn't know why she told me this, but I'm grateful that I listened, because the day after I moved everything that was important to me out of the house, construction workers working on termite damage burned it down.

What a lesson that was in listening to my guidance! When I later asked her why she didn't warn me of the fire in a way that I could have prevented it, she told me that, because I had lived and worked and raised my children in that house for thirty-one years, much of my energy was in the walls of the house, which I didn't even know could happen. She told me that I would have become ill from the people who purchased the house drawing on my energy, so Spirit wanted it to burn. Wow! Talk about keeping me safe!

My Divine guidance often tells me little things too, such as something I am forgetting to pack for a trip. It's very reassuring to experience her watching out for me. I'm constantly thanking her for all the guidance, love, and wisdom she offers me, but I know that she keeps doing this because I listen to her.

It's amazing to me how often the arrogant ego believes that it knows better than Divine guidance does. Often when I'm working with clients, they tell me what their wounded selves are saying. Then I ask them to go to their guidance and ask for the truth about that. Even though the truth that they receive from guidance makes them feel much better than what their wounded selves are telling them, they frequently don't trust it, saying, "But how can I be sure this is true?"

"How does it make you feel?"

"Great! But maybe I'm just making it up."

"How do you know you are not making up what your wounded self is telling you that is making you feel bad?"

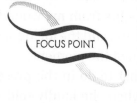
FOCUS POINT

When you trust that your wounded feelings are telling you that you are off track in your thinking and behavior and that the thoughts and images from your guidance that make you feel peaceful within are telling you that you are on track, then you will begin to feel so much safer and empowered in your life!

Half of trusting your guidance is trusting your feelings — your inner guidance. Remember, your guidance speaks to you through your feelings (your soul within) and through thoughts and images that pop into your mind from your higher soul, which is all around you.

"The fact that it makes you feel great is letting you know that it is the truth," I tell my clients. When you trust that your wounded feelings are telling you that you are off track in your thinking and behavior and that the thoughts and images from your guidance that make you feel peaceful within are telling you that you are on track, then you will begin to feel much safer and empowered in your life!

Fears of Opening to Your Guidance

- "I'm afraid if I open to my guidance, I will be told that I have to do something I don't want to do."
- "When I think about opening to God, I feel terrified, like I will just vanish."
- "I'm afraid that if I stop my self-judgments and open to guidance, I will lose my motivation."
- "I'm afraid if I open to learning about love with my guidance, I will be weak and easily taken advantage of."
- "I'm afraid if I open to guidance, I will discover that there is nothing there, that I am truly alone."

These are comments I often hear from clients who are struggling with connecting to their guidance. Where does all this fear come from?

The wounded self is naturally terrified of letting go to guidance. This part of us is terrified that if we open to our guidance, we will lose ourselves. But the truth is that we will gain ourselves — our true selves.

Examples of what really happens when you open up to your guidance follow:

- You will become aware of what you want to do — what brings you joy.
- You will discover who you really are. You will discover your essence, your true, core soul self. And the energy of the wounded self does not vanish. This energy, which has creatively managed to get you through your life so far, is now available for true creativity.
- You will be filled with creativity and aliveness. You might be doing

the same work, but now it is not from fear or the need for approval but to express who you are. Rather than being less motivated, you become more motivated to fully express all that you are.

- You move into your true power — the power to take loving care of yourself and to speak up for yourself. When you open to guidance and discover the incredible being that you are, you no longer need others' approval to feel worthy and lovable. As a result, you no longer need to try to control others by giving yourself up.
- You will discover that you are never alone. You will discover that your guidance is always here. It is always supporting you in your highest good and always letting you know each moment when you are thinking and behaving in ways that support your highest good as well as when you are off course.

When you choose to open to guidance, there is a loss, but it is not of your true self. In the moments when you surrender, you gain your self — your power, joy, peace, and ability to manifest your dreams. What you lose in moments of true surrender are your fear, anxiety, depression, guilt, shame, anger, judgment, insecurity, and illusion of control. Is this really a loss?

The Path of Love

Many people claim to be devoted to spiritual paths, yet love does not seem to be a part of their quests. What are they doing that they claim is spiritual if learning about loving themselves and others is not their highest priority?

- Some people attempt to use religion and prayer as a form of control — hoping to have control over getting what they want if they pray "right" or believe the "right" thing. Often, they are very judgmental toward others who don't believe as they do, which certainly has nothing to do with love.
- Some people use prayer and meditation as an addiction — a way to bliss out and avoid responsibility for their feelings, which is called a spiritual bypass.
- Some people believe that being selfless and just giving to others is the path of love. But without loving themselves and sharing their love from a full place within, they might have an agenda of getting

others' love — or getting God's love — attached to their selfless-
ness. Anything we do with this kind of agenda is a form of control.
- Some people are fascinated with things like learning to leave their
bodies or the power of crystals and precious stones, and they forget that the important part of the spiritual path is about love.
- Some people spend years studying spiritual literature, such as the
Bible, and they have all the knowledge in their minds but none
in their experience. They believe that knowledge rather than the
actual devotion to loving themselves and others will somehow get
them where they want to go.

When you make learning about love your highest priority — more
important than getting love or avoiding pain or feeling safe — you
will eat well and take loving care of yourself in all ways. This is when
your frequency will be high enough to easily connect with your Divine
guidance.

Once you have the information of the truth and the loving action,
then you're ready to move into step 5 of Inner Bonding.

CHAPTER 17

INNER BONDING STEP 5: TAKE LOVING ACTION

Simon, an Inner Bonding participant, said the following: "I've had incredible moments of connection and grace of late, as well as synchronicity and oneness, and I've felt so incredibly grateful that Inner Bonding came into my life. I feel like it's the best thing that ever happened to me.

"When it came into my life, I was looking for something to make me feel better, but now I realize that's only the start. The path Inner Bonding puts you on is way more profound and meaningful than I could ever have possibly imagined. I feel it has completely changed my view of life, the universe, and much more besides, and it gets deeper and deeper and deeper.

"Obviously there are lows still, but I'm trying to welcome them, and I feel like I learn and grow each time they come. Working from 'in to out' has such a powerful effect on the world around you; it's really magical."

Step 5 of Inner Bonding is taking the loving action you learned in step 4. Healing is about moving from your false belief system into living in truth. It's about moving beyond judgment and into compassion for all your feelings. It's about forgiveness for all mistakes you and others have made — for being humans and doing the best we could at the time, given our level of understanding. It's about taking loving action for yourself and others.

While bringing through the truth from your spiritual guidance (step 4) is essential in healing your false beliefs, it is not enough. Nor is it enough to gain understanding and release your old pain and fear. Unless you, as a loving adult, take new loving action for yourself, nothing really changes — nothing heals. For example, if your daughter came to you and told you she was scared of your yelling and you listened and understood but made no attempt to change your behavior, your child would not feel heard or loved. Likewise, if your inner child is hungry for love, compassion, connection, attention, safe boundaries, the end of an intolerable situation at work, a fit-and-healthy body, or simply more fun and you listen and understand but take no action, your inner child will continue to feel unloved, unlovable, alone, and unfulfilled. And your wounded self will continue to protect against these painful feelings with various addictions.

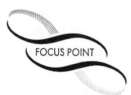

FOCUS POINT

While bringing through the truth from your spiritual guidance is essential in healing false beliefs, it is not enough. Unless you, as a loving adult, take new loving action on your own behalf, nothing really changes.

You can tell yourself the truth all day, staring into the mirror and affirming over and over that you are a beautiful, wonderful child of God, but if you do not treat yourself as a beautiful, wonderful child of God, your inner child will not believe your affirmations. Words mean very little without action. A loving adult takes action on the inner child's behalf.

Do you recall the story of my client Hannah, the woman who binged on cookies and the like because at times she felt very empty inside? (See chapter 9.) The first thing I did with Hannah was ask her to imagine a spiritual source to turn to and to ask this source to embrace her.

Hannah immediately imagined her grandfather, whom she had dearly loved as a child but who had died when she was five. She said she had often felt her grandfather around her, but she had never thought to turn to him for help. Now, as she imagined him holding her, she began to cry with the joy of feeling his love for her.

"While your grandfather is holding you, imagine the empty part of you that wants to overeat," I suggested. "Imagine that you are holding her while your grandfather is holding you. Ask her to describe how you are treating her and why it causes her to feel so empty."

Over the days and weeks that followed, Hannah's deeper self, her authentic being, began revealing the truth of her situation to her. To sum up the insight that came to her, it's as if her true self was saying to her, "The thing you always do that I just hate is to go along with everything Bernard wants. What he needs and feels are always more important to you than I am. You don't speak up for me. Ever since we married him, it's like Bernard is supposed to make me happy instead of you making me happy. I need you to make me happy by taking care of me instead of taking care of Bernard so that he'll love us. I need you to love me."

As Hannah tapped into her loving essence, she healed her empty, alone feelings, which led to the gradual vanishing of her binge eating.

Sometimes taking loving action is hard. Richard, another client, was having a hard time taking loving action: "I know that taking action is a big area of weakness for me. What do you think helps most to strengthen and develop the loving adult? Is being loving just a choice driven by willpower? Does it take hitting bottom before we finally muster the fortitude? I'm obviously struggling in this area."

I explained that it's not a matter of willpower, nor do we need to hit bottom to muster the fortitude to take loving action. I remember the day, many years ago, when I was struggling with the same issue. I was also struggling with why I was even on the planet and wondering about the purpose of life. Taking loving action seemed like a Herculean effort. I can recall the exact moment all that changed for me. While I was sitting cross-legged on my bed feeling lost and alone, it occurred to me to ask my Divine guidance about this issue. The guidance I needed came back quickly and clearly:

"The purpose of life is to evolve in your ability to love. This has to start with learning to love yourself. You are a spark of the whole, which is God that is love. 'God that is love' isn't a static entity. The energy of love that is God is ever evolving. As you evolve in your ability to love, so God evolves."

I was blown away by this insight. I knew in my heart and soul that what my guidance was telling me was true. I could feel the truth of it throughout my whole being. I began to see that I was on the planet to evolve in my ability to love, which involved learning to fully manifest the gifts I had been given. I realized I could do this only when I recognized and came to deeply cherish the essence of who I am, the spark of the Divine that is my core.

When we know how magnificent we are and how magnificent the essence of each of us is, we find ourselves spontaneously motivated to love ourselves and share our love. By deeply valuing my soul, I became highly motivated to take loving action for myself and others. When you see the beauty of who you truly are, it's far easier to want to be loving toward yourself and to take loving action for yourself. The more you do this, the more filled with love you become and the more you naturally share love with others.

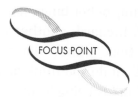

FOCUS POINT

When you see the beauty of who you truly are, you want to be loving to and take loving action for yourself. The more you do this, the more filled with love you become, and the more you share love with others.

You Need to See, Love, and Value Yourself to Feel Divine Love

To illustrate the importance of taking loving action for yourself, I want to share with you a conversation I had with a client. I'll use the term "God" since this is what my client used. Let me clarify that to experience the love we speak of in this dialogue, it's not necessary to believe in God; however, you do need to learn how to access the spiritual center within you and all around you from which this love flows.

My client Tracey began our session by asking, "When I open myself to my spiritual guidance, aren't I supposed to feel loved by God?"

"Yes," I answered, "but you might have a misconception about how you experience this love. When do you feel love in your heart?"

"I feel the most love when I'm playing with my nephews," Tracey responded.

"So when you play with your nephews, your heart is open, right?"

"Yes. I love them so much that naturally I enjoy playing with them."

"Well, this is what it feels like to feel God's love," I explained. "When your intention is to love, your heart opens and floods with Divine love. The same will occur when your intent is to love yourself. Can you imagine loving yourself the way you love your nephews?"

"I think that's a problem for me," Tracey admitted. "It's easy for me to show them love and attention, but it's hard to do this for myself."

"Why do you think this is?" I asked.

"It doesn't feel worth going to all the trouble."

"So if you had a daughter who was just like you were as a child, would you say she wasn't worth loving?"

"I would never say that," Tracey was quick to respond. "I would love loving her!"

"This is why you don't feel God's love for you. To feel the love, your heart needs to be open. When you are in your wounded self and judging yourself as unworthy of love, your heart is closed. To feel the love that is God, you have to want to love yourself and open to learning about what is loving to you. Right now, take a deep breath and focus inside. What are you feeling?"

"I feel somewhat anxious," Tracey confessed.

I suggested, "Take a moment to ask your deeper self what you are telling her right now that's causing her to feel anxious."

Tracey reported that she was telling herself she had to do this "right."

I responded, "When you put pressure on yourself to do it right, you feel anxious. The anxiety is your inner guidance letting you know that you're telling yourself a lie. Remember, your feelings (anxiety, depression, anger, guilt, and shame) let you know you are off track in your thinking. They let you know that your true self is feeling abandoned. I suggest you ask your guidance, 'Is it true that my worth depends on doing something right?'"

After a few moments Tracey said, "I'm realizing how sweet and kind my true self is, even when she doesn't do something right."

"Can you embrace her for her sweetness and kindness right

now?" I proposed. "Can you hold her in love, bringing her into your heart?"

"Yes, I can!" Tracey enthused.

After another short silence, I inquired, "How does that feel?"

"It feels great! I'm actually having sensations of warmth and peace in my heart."

"Because you are loving yourself, you are feeling God's love for you," I confirmed.

"I think I'm getting this," Tracey said. "I can't feel God's love for me when I'm not loving myself. When I criticize myself and put pressure on myself to do everything right, I can't feel God's love because my heart is closed to it. But when I love myself, I feel God's love for me."

Taking loving action means learning to love both the core self and the wounded self. But we can't love the wounded self until we notice it. Only when we're willing to notice ourselves acting out the needs of our ego — and do so without judging ourselves — will we be able to make new, loving choices. We need to release all criticism and accept the angry, hurt, ashamed, and frightened parts of ourselves with love and compassion.

Why have compassion for our wounded selves? Because our egos have quite simply been doing the best they could to take care of us and help us feel safe. Loving yourself means understanding and having compassion for all the parts of you that you might have hated or judged as inadequate, unlovable, and unworthy. You will recover from your addictions when you learn to be loving to both your core self and your wounded self.

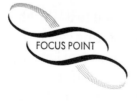

FOCUS POINT

We need to release all criticism and accept the angry, hurt, ashamed, and frightened parts of ourselves with love and compassion. Loving ourselves means understanding and having compassion for all the parts of ourselves that we might have hated or judged as inadequate, unlovable, and unworthy.

The Power of Gratitude for Your Essence

Loving action comes from an open heart, and as I previously stated, gratitude is one of the quickest ways to open the heart. The most powerful feelings of gratitude are feelings that arise in the present moment: for your soul, your body, the people in your life whom you love and who love you, the animals you love and who love you, the guidance of Spirit, and the very fact of your life. Also powerful are feelings of gratitude for big and small acts of kindness, understanding, caring, gentleness, and tenderness — for loved ones and strangers — and for new insights that open your heart.

Remember to express gratitude for the things that nurture you — healthy food, a hot bath, a wonderful book, the beauty of nature, a belly laugh, moving music, a great movie, a cuddly pet, a child's laughter, a tender hug, and time with friends and loved ones.

My client Maddy had been practicing Inner Bonding for about eighteen months. She had attended a number of intensives and was sitting with me in an advanced intensive. She had been doing really well staying connected with herself and with her guidance, and she had experienced times of peace and joy that she had never felt before. Suddenly, all her progress seemed to vanish, and she was back in her major addiction — trying to control a man.

She and Erik had recently connected in a way that she had not connected with anyone before, but after only a couple of months, it seemed to her that he was pulling away. She found herself obsessing about him and unable to sleep when she didn't hear from him.

"Maddy, what made you fall for Erik?"

"He thought I was wonderful. I felt seen and cherished like never before."

"What are you not seeing or cherishing about yourself? What are you telling yourself that makes you feel as if you are not wonderful?"

The answer was not immediately apparent. Maddy had done a lot of work on herself and was valuing herself like she had never done before, which is why she was so perplexed by her obsessive thinking about Erik. After doing some searching and finally opening to learning with her higher self, she got in touch with what she had been saying to herself: "You will never get what you want because you don't deserve it. You will never be good enough."

No wonder Erik's seeing and cherishing her felt like manna from heaven! On a deep, unconscious level, Maddy was almost constantly shaming and blaming herself whenever anything went wrong. Her inner child felt anything but seen and cherished by her.

"I don't get this," she said. "I know I'm a good person, so I don't get why I still feel this way."

"Do you ever feel deep gratitude for your soul — for the good, kind, caring, compassionate, creative, loving soul that you are?"

She looked surprised. "I've never thought of feeling grateful for my soul. Now that you say it, I've often felt extremely grateful for my kids, but never for the child in me — my own soul."

"Can you find the place in you that feels grateful for your children and bring that same feeling to your inner child?"

"Yes, I can do that!"

"How do you feel when you do that?"

"I feel wonderful, just as good, if not better, than when Erik thinks I'm wonderful!"

That evening Maddy and Erik had a close and connected conversation, the best in a long time. It was obvious to Maddy that because she had been abandoning herself and making Erik responsible for her sense of worth, he had been feeling pulled at and overwhelmed, and he had pulled away. As a result of her seeing and cherishing her soul and feeling deep gratitude for the beauty that she is, she no longer pulled on him to give her what she was not giving to herself.

Along with gratitude, the beauty of art, music, and nature can open your heart. Beauty and gratitude are food for the soul. Equally powerful are compassion for your and others' feelings and situations and forgiveness for yourself and others. Compassion and forgiveness are balms to the soul.

Without Loving Action, Intention Means Nothing

The gift of being able to choose our intentions is one of the greatest we have been given — the gift of free will. Choosing, moment by moment, the intention to learn and love or the intention to protect against pain is the most powerful choice we have in life — the one that makes the most difference.

However, as I've previously stated, intention can be subtle. We might think we are choosing the intent to love ourselves and others, but if loving action does not follow, then we have not truly chosen the intention to learn and love.

A true intention to love propels us into loving action. If you do not take the loving action, then you need to be honest with yourself: You were not intent on loving yourself and others. When your intention is a deep and abiding desire to be more loving with yourself and others, it will fuel the loving actions you need to take. Choosing that intention is vital to eventually taking the loving actions.

For example, if you have a true and deep desire to be healthy and fit and to have a high enough frequency to connect with your Divine guidance, what will you do? What loving actions will you take? You will read many books on health and nutrition. You will stop eating sugar and other junk foods and start eating clean, organic foods. You will stay tuned in to your body to learn how different foods affect you. You will begin a consistent exercise program. You will practice Inner Bonding to deal with stress and bring about inner peace. These and other loving actions would naturally follow from your deep desire to be healthy and to connect with your Divine guidance.

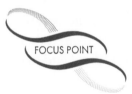

FOCUS POINT

When your intention is a deep and abiding desire to be more loving with yourself and others, it will fuel the loving actions you need to take.

However, if you *say* you want to be healthy and connected but you do not take these loving actions, then you need to be honest with yourself that something is more important than being healthy and fit, which is to continue to protect against pain with your various addictions. The lack of loving action indicates that being healthy, fit, and divinely connected is not your highest priority. When you have a deep intention to love yourself, loving actions always follow.

Loving Actions in Relationship Challenges

How much of your behavior is in reaction to your partner? Consider how you feel when your partner

- gets angry or irritated with you
- withdraws from you
- blames or judges you

- misunderstands you or does not see you accurately
- does not take time for you
- complains, behaves needy, or pouts
- threatens you physically, financially, emotionally, or sexually
- threatens the relationship or behaves in ways that feel as if he or she is rejecting to you

Do you react in one of the following ways? You might
- explain, defend
- shame, judge
- comply
- withdraw, shut down, ignore, resist
- yell, blame, attack
- complain
- cry as a victim
- go into the fight, flight, or freeze response

These reactions either escalate the conflict or create a tense distance between partners. All these reactions stem from a desire to have control over getting love or avoiding pain, but they tend to create the very situations that you are trying to avoid.

When people fall in love, they fall in love with each other's essence. But as they get deeper into the relationship, their fears of rejection and engulfment are triggered, and they move into the protective, controlling behavior of their wounded selves. This can cause conflict, and there are only two possible loving actions in conflict: (1) State your truth without shame or blame, and move into an intention to learn with the other person, sharing and caring about each other's very good reasons for believing or acting as you are. (2) If the other person isn't open to learning with you, then state your truth and lovingly disengage.

Lovingly disengaging is very different from withdrawing. When you withdraw, your heart is closed, and you are punishing the other person with your withdrawal of love. When you lovingly disengage, you move out of range of a situation that might be hurtful to you. You are not angry. You let the other person know that you will be back in thirty minutes to see whether he or she is open to learning. Then you do your inner work to keep your heart open in order to not take the other's behavior personally and to lovingly manage any painful feelings of loneliness, heartache, and helplessness concerning the other person.

In thirty minutes, you check back to see whether the other person is open. If he or she doesn't open, then you need to open to learning with your Divine guidance about how to take loving care of yourself in the face of the other person being closed. Trying to resolve a conflict when one or both of you are closed won't get you anywhere. However, you will find that conflicts are easy to resolve when both of you are open to learning about yourselves and each other.

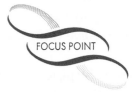

FOCUS POINT

Conflicts are easy to resolve when you and your partner are open to learning about yourselves and each other.

Attempts to get others to open up are generally met with resistance. In fact, trying to get them to do so, even with kindness, is just another form of control. Most people who want to control also don't wish to be controlled and will resist when they feel someone is attempting to control them, even if it's just to get them to open up.

When you feel you are open to learning and the other person isn't, the key to not causing more problems is to accept your helplessness over the other's intention. If you completely accept that there's nothing you can do to get others to listen to you, understand you, agree with you, or accept you, you won't pursue the discussion. You'll stop banging your head against the wall when it's obvious there's no hope of the wall coming down, and then you will focus on the loving actions you need to do for yourself.

We all have a strong tendency to convince ourselves that if we just say the right things in just the right way or do the right things, the other will finally hear us and care about what we feel and want. Because of this illusion, we can exhaust ourselves in fruitless arguments that leave us more frustrated and lonely than ever.

Rather than arguing, lecturing, pleading, crying, or blaming in an attempt to change the other person's intention, it's far more loving to ourselves and the other to disengage from combative discussions until both parties are open. As I stated, it's important to be aware that walking away can also be a form of control if the intent of walking away is to punish the other person by withholding your love. The energy you will have if you walk away in anger and blame is entirely different from the energy of disengaging because it's the loving thing to do for yourself and for the other person. When you walk away as a loving adult, you can simply say, "Let's give this some space and talk about it later." Do not say, "Let's talk about this later, when you are open."

In my workshops and intensives, when I state that it's more loving to walk away from a combative situation than to continue to argue, someone invariably comments, "When I walk away, my partner often says, 'You always run away rather than stay and resolve things.' How would you respond to this?"

If someone blames you for taking a loving action by peacefully disengaging, the person is still trying to control you. He or she hopes to hook you back in. The wisest move — the loving action toward yourself — is not to respond because anything you say will be taken as a defense, and you'll be right back in the fray. Yes, I know this takes practice, but it's worth the effort.

Learning and taking loving action must begin with ourselves, especially with learning to love ourselves, since the intention to learn about loving ourselves is essential for our development as well as for our Divine connection. This is also the basis for creating loving relationships. On the other hand, self-abandonment, which is the opposite of loving ourselves and taking loving action for ourselves, is the major cause of not only spiritual disconnection but also of relationship failure.

Conflict resolution is not just about solving a problem. It is about using the problem to learn about and heal the deeper issues of self-abandonment that are generally the underlying cause of the conflict. This is what leads to growth and healing. Relationships offer us the most powerful arena for personal and spiritual growth. They are the PhD of growth and healing!

Eating Well in Your Relationship

Shopping and cooking for one person is one thing. You decide what you want, buy it, and prepare it. It's when you introduce a second person that things can get complicated — fast. I have come across no small number of couples who say they are open to living in a manner that promotes health and well-being, yet it never seems to happen in practice. Usually one party wants to do something about his or her eating habits, and the other proves to be recalcitrant. This tends to result in the relationship becoming stuck. Sometimes eating and drinking issues lead to the relationship's end.

In any interaction with another person, there are always two levels of communication: intent and content. Intent refers to your deepest desire — what is most important to you in the moment. Content is the issue you may be discussing, such as time, money, tasks, communication, sexuality, parenting, relationships with family and friends, food, health, and so on. The content is the topic, and the intent is the container you interact within.

Discussions over content degenerate into arguments when one or both parties operate from the intent to control. As I stated earlier, issues can't be resolved unless both intend to learn. On the contrary, even more problems arise when we choose control rather than learning because now the controlling behavior becomes an issue to fight over.

My client Karen has been married to Chris for forty years. Now in their sixties, they are experiencing health problems. In his younger years, before he married, Chris was devoted to purchasing organic foods. Karen, on the other hand, said she believed in eating healthily but never got around to purchasing organics, claiming they were "ridiculously expensive."

In the early years of their marriage, whenever they went shopping, which most of the time they did together, this couple argued over the issue. Chris constantly urged, "Let's get the organic kind. It's so much healthier." But as their cart rolled up to the checkout, it was evident that Karen had put her foot down yet again, and Chris gave in to avoid an argument.

Over the years, even though money was never a problem for them, Chris continued to capitulate to his economizing wife. He would protest, even sulk on occasion, but that was the extent of his stand. Consequently, Karen rode roughshod over his protests. Despite the fact that today Chris is having difficulties with his health, he continues to give in to his wife instead of following his intention to eat organically — something he could have opted to do long ago regardless of how she eats and without trying to control her.

The irony is that if you were to ask Karen about their diet, she'd tell you they eat incredibly healthily. But in reality, she never checks package contents, always opts for the cheapest deal, and hasn't read any of the books or articles Chris has given her regarding health throughout their marriage.

The fact is, neither Karen nor Chris is open to walk the path to robust health. Both are intent on protecting rather than learning.

The Power of Safe Touch

Learning to love yourself creates the inner safety and connection with self and Spirit that is an absolutely necessary aspect of healing. There is another necessary aspect — safety and connection with another.

We don't heal alone. The steps of Inner Bonding are powerful, and they are essential for being able to be open enough to connect with others, but they do not replace connection and safety with another. Our deepest wounds occurred in our relationships as we were growing up, and we need others to heal these wounds. While others cannot do it for us, they can do it with us.

Instead of reaching for food or drink or some other pacifying addiction when we are in pain, it can be helpful to reach for touch from another living being — as long as it's done in an informed, conscious way. The right sort of loving touch will awaken our loving essence, which increasingly blossoms, helping to heal the pain that drives our addictions. In fact, research indicates that receiving safe, unconditionally loving touch and holding is one of the most powerful ways of healing trauma.

Were you deprived of comforting touch as a child? I was. My mother held me, but her touch was so needy and engulfing that I hated being held or touched by her.

To know they are loved and to help them learn to regulate their feelings, babies and toddlers need warm, tender, comforting touch. Without this loving touch, they feel rejected, which becomes part of their emotional template. If the deprivation continues long enough, they feel utterly abandoned — a horrific feeling that will define them for years to come unless they are awakened to their need for bonding with their lost selves.

As babies coming into the world, we need to feel safe and loved. We need to be held and carried by a loving adult during most of our waking hours. Our basic needs should be met quickly — our need for food, diaper changes, and smiles, as well as comfort when we're lonely or our bodies are giving us a hard time. We need to sleep next to a loving parent. In most indigenous societies, this is exactly what happens. Thankfully, this kind of parenting is more common today, but it was rare in our society when I was born.

Were your parents loving adults, capable of giving love to themselves, each other, and you? Or were they needy, anxious, overwhelmed, angry, or depressed? When they held you, did they bring love to you, or did you feel smothered by them? If you were a child who didn't like being held by one or the other of your parents or caregivers, there's a good possibility your mother or father or caregiver was needy and tried to get love from you instead of give love to you.

Were you fed when you were hungry, or were you put on a schedule? Were you held, or were you left alone in a crib or playpen? When you cried, did someone come, or did you end up crying for a long time and finally giving up? Did you sleep near or with your parents, or were you left alone? Were you treated with tenderness and caring, or was there abuse?

Many try to quench their neediness through sex, but this is not at all what the deeper self is crying out for. In fact, sexualizing the need for touch can cause sexual acting out or sexual addiction. It's like trying to satisfy thirst with salt water; it will never give you what you truly need.

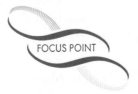

FOCUS POINT

Sexualizing the need for touch can cause sexual acting out or sexual addiction. It's like trying to satisfy thirst with salt water; it will never give you what you truly need.

Leticia consulted me because she had a hard time connecting with people. Having been abused and neglected as a child by her single mother, she had never experienced a sense of bonding with another person.

Aware of her deep longing to be held and physically nurtured by a woman, she decided that she needed to be in a relationship with a woman. Although she had become sexually involved with a woman in the hopes of fulfilling the longing, it wasn't helping her, which left her feeling confused.

"Why is it when Gayle holds me, it doesn't heal that longing in me?" she asked.

"What generally happens when Gayle holds you?" I inquired.

"We end up making love."

"So is your longing a longing for sex, or is it a longing for being lovingly held?"

"I really want the holding," Leticia said. "I also want to be nursed. I thought if she nursed me, that deep longing would go away. But it hasn't, and I don't understand why."

I thought for a moment, then inquired, "When you were a baby and needed to be held, did you also need sex?"

"No!" Leticia said adamantly. "Why would you think that?"

"I have my reasons," I assured her. "Just follow my line of inquiry for the moment. If someone had held you as a baby, then been sexual with you, would that have been loving to you?"

"Ugh. No, absolutely not!"

"Well, it's no different today. The imprint from the time you were a baby wants you to have what you didn't receive. You want to be held with love, a longing that's emanating from your authentic self as it seeks to come fully alive. When you are held with love and then have sex, it's as if you are being violated. It isn't love; it's a betrayal. Do you see why it isn't helping? You are trying to heal what happened to you as a baby with an adult activity, which can never work. If you want a sexual relationship with either a man or a woman, look for that. But if you want to be nurtured, you need to find a totally different kind of relationship."

Looking utterly surprised by this insight, Leticia blurted out, "So does this mean I might not want to be in a relationship with a woman?"

"Wanting to be held has nothing to do with your sexuality. The issue here is whether you are more sexually attracted to men or to women."

Leticia didn't hesitate in her response. "To men. I've had much better sex with men than with Gayle."

"Then it seems you've sexualized your need for being held."

"So what do I do now?"

"Finding appropriate touch is unfortunately not always easy. If you have a good friend or relative who can hold you with tenderness and love, that is great. You could also come to one of my Inner Bonding intensives and receive a lot of safe holding. But while these steps can be helpful, the most important thing you can do for yourself is to open up to your essential being, which will bring you spiritual guidance in terms of how you relate to others as well as supply the ongoing love we all need."

Leticia was fortunate. She had a motherly friend, a woman with children of her own, who was more than happy to hold her. Over the months of being held by her friend, her longing gradually diminished.

Loving touch comes from a place within that doesn't need anything back. Touch serves as a conduit for the love that is the nature of the Divine. This is the touch we need, the kind that says, "You matter. You have value. You are a beautiful child of the universe, and I am blessed to be able to be a conduit of love for you."

It has become common in Western society to hug, often even the first time we meet someone. It's therefore important to recognize that there are hugs and then there are "hugs." Genuinely loving hugs have no element of neediness to them, only a welcoming and valuing of the other. In contrast, needy hugs — including those with inappropriate sexual overtones — always "suck." There's a world of difference between these kinds of hugs.

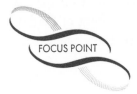

FOCUS POINT

Loving touch comes from a place within that doesn't need anything back.

I'm an affectionate person. Because my mother's hugs were needy and after I turned twelve my father's hugs became sexual, by the time

I started dating, I was so starved for hugs that I often found myself in difficult situations. While what I wanted was caring hugs, what I mostly got was needy and often sexual hugs from the boys I dated. It was some years before I could differentiate the energetic difference between nurturing hugs and needy or inappropriate, sexual hugs.

It's important to become discerning. We've seen that when people aren't in touch with their essence, they experience an emptiness that acts as a vacuum as it tries to suck love out of others. It's an attempt to get the love they aren't experiencing within themselves. While needy huggers might have warm smiles on their faces, the energy behind the hug doesn't feel good. If you tune in to the energy, you'll know instantly that the person hugging you is trying to take from you rather than give to you or share with you. You can also tell when you are hugging someone in this way.

With inappropriate sexual hugs, the hugger is trying to be filled through sexual energy. I experience this a lot with many, but not all, of the men I meet. Occasionally I meet a man who hugs from a heart full of love. What a gift it is to be hugged by a truly loving man or woman!

Before I understood this, I allowed myself to be taken from, and it felt awful, but I didn't know how to take loving action for myself. Now I deal with this very differently. I understand that the pull is from the other person's undeveloped essence, and I feel compassion for the person. Then instead of allowing myself to be taken from, I freely give my love to the aspect of them that was crushed and left undeveloped all those years ago. This feels much better to me than pulling away, and I also don't end up feeling used. I even reached a place where I was able to hug my mother and give my love to her undeveloped center.

Healthy touch is what loving parents who are connected with themselves and their spiritual source give to their children. Their children are truly blessed to receive this love, for it's a part of the foundation of their sense of worth and a vital aspect of learning to regulate their feelings, which will have an impact on every aspect of their future health.

The Lessons of Loneliness

What might it look like to embrace your power? Imagine you feel full of love. You enjoy your own company immensely, so much so that you want to share the wonderful person you are with other wonderful people. But when you seek to connect with someone — a partner, a friend, or an acquaintance — the experience gives rise to a sense of loneliness. Instead of allowing this to become about you, you might want to recognize that the feeling of loneliness is telling you that the person is closed. This is important information because instead of trying to create a relationship with someone incapable of connecting, you can now take loving care of yourself by finding some other way to express your love.

Can you accept your helplessness when it comes to getting another person to connect with you? Can you see that not forcing the issue or turning tail and sulking about it honors their right to be unique, alone in their uniqueness like we are? Others' unloving behavior toward us isn't something to fight against but something to accept. When we finally accept it, then we are free to take loving actions for ourselves.

The experience of being alone — not the aloneness that comes from self-abandonment, but being alone because no one is around — is completely transformed once we learn to manage it rather than avoid it. Actually, "manage" is an inadequate term, since it's only a first step toward what can become a blissful state — a mode of being that arises from within as we learn to embrace our lovability and relish our uniqueness.

This is because once we rediscover the identity we lost touch with long ago, we *love* being who we are. We like our own company because we experience being who we are as a joyous thing. This in turn enables us to enjoy others for who they are and not because we need them to assuage empty feelings inside ourselves. As pointed out earlier, the empty feeling is different from feeling lonely, the one coming from self-abandonment and the other being entirely natural when we want to connect with others and no one is available.

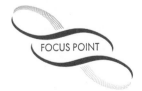

FOCUS POINT

Once we rediscover the identity we lost touch with long ago, we love being who we are.

When we're connected to who we are in our heart of hearts, our souls, we don't feel alone inside when we are alone for a time. Having no one to share friendship with, to love, or to love us — because either there's no one around or those around us are closed to a meaningful connection with us — can be a lonely experience, but it doesn't need to cause us despair once we know who we are. We might even find that we can be alone for long periods and, though we experience loneliness, not be damaged psychologically. Feeling lonely isn't something to critique or apologize for. It's something we simply need to accept when it occurs.

Once you take whatever loving action you were guided to take, then move into step 6 — evaluation.

CHAPTER 18

INNER BONDING STEP 6: EVALUATE YOUR ACTION

Cheryl, an InnerBonding.com member, shared the following: "I could not be moving through a recent, very painful relationship breakup with the tenderness and love I feel for myself without the practice of Inner Bonding, the online classes that I have taken, and the support of the Inner Bonding community. I cannot express the depth of gratitude I have for the work of Drs. Paul and Chopich in bringing this transformative healing path to the world."

Step 6 of the Inner Bonding process is to evaluate the effectiveness of your action. Once you have taken action, you need to evaluate whether you actually took a loving action and whether the action is working for you. In a sense, step 6 is like step 1 in that you tune inside and ask yourself how you are feeling.

Breathe into your body and notice your feelings. If you're feeling some relief, more peace inside, and some lightness, then you know that you've taken a loving action. Again, your feelings inform you.

Taking loving action often brings about an instant sense of

relief — not the kind of relief you feel when you smoke a cigarette or eat a donut or have sex, but the kind of deep inner relief that comes from being seen, understood, and loved. Do you feel happier, less alone, and more connected with yourself, others, and your Divine guidance? Is your feeling of shame diminishing? Do you feel freer and less afraid? Are you less interested in pursuing your substance or process addictions? Do you have a greater sense of personal power and self-worth? Are you feeling more playful and more creative? Are you laughing more? Are you more compassionate?

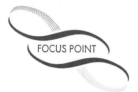

Breathe into your body and notice your feelings. If you feel some relief, more peace inside, and some lightness, then you know you've taken a loving action.

If the answers to your self-evaluation show you that healing is not happening, go back to step 4, and ask your Divine guidance to help you discover another loving action. For example, perhaps you need to speak up for yourself with someone, or you need more time in prayer. Maybe you need help with your healing process. Perhaps you need to be held by someone who can bring through unconditional love and help heal the old abandonment wound. Maybe you need to spend more time having fun with others, or you might need more time alone to pursue passions or hobbies.

Here are some questions that you, as a loving adult, can keep asking your inner child. Be sure to listen carefully to the answers. Remember, this is a process so, for example, if you ask your inner child whether he or she feels loved by you, the answer might be something like "more than I used to" or "sometimes but not often enough." The answers to these questions can help you determine where you are in your journey:

- "Are you feeling loved by me?"
- "Do you feel you can trust me to be there for you and not be self-indulgent when the urge to act out addictively comes up?"
- "Do you feel you can trust me to not harm others with my anger?"
- "Do you feel you can trust me to set good limits with others? Or are you still afraid I will give in to them or allow them to violate you and take advantage of you?"

- "Are you feeling safe inside, or are you still feeling alone and afraid?"
- "Am I defining your worth and lovability, or am I still allowing others to define you?"
- "Do you feel a deep sense of worth that cannot be shaken by others' disapproval, or are you still afraid of rejection?"

If you answered all these questions with a definite yes, then you might be an enlightened being! But if you were an enlightened being, you likely wouldn't be reading this book, so accept that we are all human and in the process of healing. There is no need to put pressure on yourself regarding the answers.

When you evaluate your actions, you cannot just analyze how you feel in the moment. Acting out addictively, such as overeating or taking out your anger on someone, generally feels good in the moment. That's how it became an addiction. Often, when you take a loving action, such as cutting out sugar or junk food; stopping drinking, taking drugs, or smoking; not acting out sexually; no longer taking responsibility for another's feelings; or no longer dumping your anger on others, you feel awful in the moment. Your wounded self feels frightened at having a crutch taken away. You feel deprived of something that gives you momentary pleasure, or you feel terrified of rejection and aloneness.

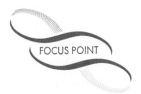

FOCUS POINT

Often, what works for you in the short term undermines you in the long term; however, what works in the long term may not feel good in the short term.

Your addictions worked to make you feel better for the moment, so when you stop them, you will likely go through a period of feeling much worse. You might go through both physical and emotional withdrawals. Often what works for you in the short term undermines you in the long term; however, what works for your best interests in the long term may not feel good in the short term.

Even though loving action may not always feel good in the moment, if it's truly in your highest good, it will feel right. You will experience a sense of integrity as you act in harmony with your soul. Lightness, freedom, and power come from taking good care of yourself, even if initially it feels difficult, frightening, or painful.

Here's the bottom line: If you look inside to evaluate your loving action and find that you are still feeling genuinely, not momentarily, depressed, frightened, hurt, angry, or powerless, then you need to go back to dialoguing with your spiritual guidance (step 4) to see what else you need to do regarding a particular situation. This process could go on for days, weeks, or sometimes even months (with very difficult issues) before you discover the loving action that really works for you regarding a particular situation. Sometimes you will need to reach out for help with this.

Experience the State of Grace

When you have been doing the six steps of Inner Bonding for a while and you are bringing through the love and giving your inner child what he or she really needs, you will find that more frequently you feel a wonderful lightness of being, a sense of fullness in your heart, and joy that bubbles up from within your soul. This is a state of grace.

Fear gradually diminishes and is replaced by peace and joy in the process of learning. The gnawing aloneness and emptiness within that led to addictive behavior no longer exists when you stay in contact with your inner child and meet his or her deep need for love through connection with your spiritual guidance. You will often feel a sense of aliveness, wholeness, integration, and even bliss.

Gradually the experience of separation from self and others that pained you so will diminish, and you will feel a sense of oneness within you and with others. You will be unwilling to behave in any way that hurts you or others; you will discover your integrity. You will experience a deep trust in yourself and your spiritual guidance. And you will discover that you no longer have to strive to believe in God, for now you know the love that is God.

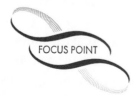

FOCUS POINT

Gradually the experience of separation from self and others that pained you so will diminish, and you will feel a sense of oneness within you and with others.

No longer will you experience others in terms of "us" and "them." There will be no judgment, no enemy. No one will be left out, and no one will be less than you or more than you, regardless of gender, race, religion, or spiritual path. You will come to understand that all ways of learning about love are valuable and all paths intended to unite with God lead to God. You will feel a deep sense of oneness with everyone and everything.

When you operate as a loving adult, you never have to wait for someone to fill your emptiness. You never have to feel alone. You have the complete freedom to fill yourself with love and peace whenever you want. You never have to wait for someone to come along to take loving action for you. You have the complete freedom to take that action for yourself. As children, we did not have this freedom. We needed others to take action for us. When they didn't, we might have become locked into thinking that we needed others to do this for us or that doing it ourselves was too much work, failing to see that taking responsibility for ourselves is a most delicious privilege and freedom.

Once you learn to take responsibility for your feelings, the way is open for you to create safe, sacred relationships. The power struggles that exist in so many relationships fall by the wayside as you learn to let go of trying to control other people and take responsibility for yourself. Conflicts get resolved in healthy ways when you learn the powerful skills of conflict resolution that are available to you.

You will experience all your relationships improving, whether or not your family, friends, or partners learn to take loving care of themselves. In addition, if you have children, as you become a loving role model of personally responsible behavior, your children will naturally learn to be personally responsible as well. Let's raise a generation of healthy children by learning how to become loving, physically healthy, spiritually connected, personally responsible adults!

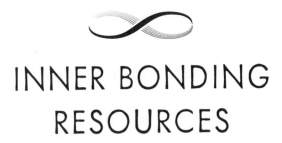

INNER BONDING
RESOURCES

For information or to schedule a phone or Skype session, please call **310-459-1700** or **888-646-6372 (888-6INNERBOND)**

Inner Bonding®, The Power to Heal Yourself: **InnerBonding.com**

Online Courses and Supplemental Inner Bonding Information
SelfQuest®
This online program teaches Inner Bonding in a very in-depth way.

Inner Bonding Facilitator Training Program
Become a certified Inner Bonding facilitator. For more information, visit www.innerbonding.com/show-page/339/ibftp.html.

Books, eBooks, Lectures, Workshops, Podcasts, Webinars
Purchase Inner Bonding courses and materials at www.innerbonding .com/store.php.

Events, Intensives, Support Groups
Learn more about Inner Bonding and about others' experiences using it at www.innerbonding.com/events.php.

Join Inner Bonding Village, **http://www.InnerBonding.com/register .php,** to receive connection and sense of community with like-minded people and caring and compassionate support for your healing and growth.

Dr. Paul's 30-Day At-Home Courses

Love Yourself
In this Inner Bonding experience, learn techniques to self-heal anxiety, depression, guilt, shame, addictions, and relationships.

Frequency
Learn methods to connect with or deepen your connection with your spiritual guidance, and learn the art of manifestation.

Loving Relationships
This home-study experience is for couples and people who seek to be partnered. Learn how to improve all your relationships.

Attracting Your Beloved
Learn how to attract the love of your life!

Passionate Purpose, Vibrant Health
Discover your passionate purpose, enhance your creativity, and create a joyful, vibrantly healthy life!

Dr. Paul's Health Resources

Cookbooks
- *Nourishing Traditions* by Sally Fallon
- *The Complete Idiot's Guide to Fermenting Foods* by Wardeh Harmon

Favorite Websites
- For sprouted organic flour and grains, go to HealthyFlour.com.
- For traditional cultures for yogurt, cheese, and sourdough bread (with excellent videos), visit CulturesforHealth.com.
- For whole-food organic supplements, see theSynergyCompany.com.

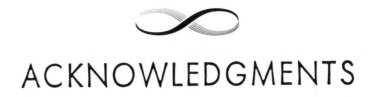

ACKNOWLEDGMENTS

Thanks to my literary agent at Waterside Productions, Johanna Maaghul, who came up with the title and supported me through the evolution of this book. Thanks to Stephen Dinan, CEO of The Shift Network, who introduced me to Waterside Productions.

Thanks to my publisher, Melody Swanson of Light Technology Publishing, for telling me she loved my book and that it would be an honor to publish it. Thanks to Monica Markley, my editor at Light Technology, for being a joy to work with.

Thanks to David Ord for putting me into his busy writing and editing schedule and working hard to help make this book so readable.

Thanks to Dr. Erika Chopich, the cocreator of Inner Bonding and my closest friend, for reading this book and giving me helpful suggestions and feedback.

I'm deeply grateful to my wonderful friend Marci Shimoff for writing the foreword; it brought me to tears. Through your love and generosity of spirit, you continue to provide miracles for all of us.

I feel very blessed by my wonderful friends and colleagues who read my book and endorsed it with their beautiful words.

Thanks to all my clients, workshop and intensive participants, and students in my online courses. I feel blessed that you show up to do your Inner Bonding work, sharing your hearts and souls with me and giving me the sacred privilege of being a "midwife" for your wholeness, peace, joy, and relationship healing. My work is my passion, and I could not do it if you didn't have the courage to show up for yourselves.

ABOUT THE AUTHOR

Dr. Margaret Paul is a best-selling author and a popular *Huffington Post* and *Mind-BodyGreen* writer. Her books have been translated into ten languages. She is the cocreator of the powerful Inner Bonding® self-healing process and the related SelfQuest® self-healing online program recommended by actress Lindsay Wagner and singer Alanis Morissette. SelfQuest is a powerful tool for emotional healing, spiritual growth, healing relationship issues, healing addictions, and developing personal responsibility in life and work.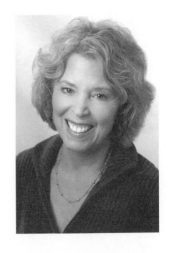

Dr. Paul holds a PhD in psychology and has appeared on numerous radio and television shows, including *Oprah*. Dr. Paul has been counseling people individually and as couples since 1968, and she has been leading groups, teaching classes and workshops, and working with partnerships and businesses since 1973. She is passionate about evolving and teaching the process of Inner Bonding by administering her popular website, InnerBonding.com.

Dr. Paul has three children and three grandchildren. In her spare time, she is an artist.

TO ORDER PRINT BOOKS
Visit LightTechnology.com, Call 928-526-1345 or 1-800-450-0985,
or Check Amazon.com or Your Favorite Bookstore

BOOKS THROUGH DRUNVALO MELCHIZEDEK

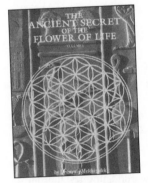

THE ANCIENT SECRET OF THE FLOWER OF LIFE, VOLUME 1

Also available in Spanish as *Antiguo Secreto Flor de la Vida, Volumen 1*

Once, all life in the universe knew the Flower of Life as the creation pattern, the geometrical design leading us into and out of physical existence. Then from a very high state of consciousness, we fell into darkness, and the secret was hidden for thousands of years, encoded in the cells of all life.

$25.00 • 240 PP. • Softcover • ISBN 978-1-891824-17-3

THE ANCIENT SECRET OF THE FLOWER OF LIFE, VOLUME 2

Also available in Spanish as *Antiguo Secreto Flor de la Vida, Volumen 2*

Drunvalo shares the instructions for the Mer-Ka-Ba meditation, step-by-step techniques for the re-creation of the energy field of the evolved human, which is the key to ascension and the next dimensional world. If done from love, this ancient process of breathing prana opens up for us a world of tantalizing possibility in this dimension, from protective powers to the healing of oneself, others, and even the planet.

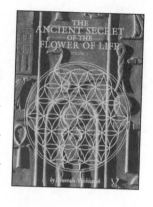

$25.00 • 272 PP. • Softcover • ISBN 978-1-891824-21-0

LIVING IN THE HEART

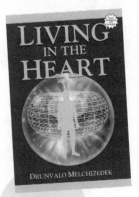

Also available in Spanish as *Viviendo en el Corazón*

"Long ago we humans used a form of communication and sensing that did not involve the brain in any way; rather, it came from a sacred place within our hearts. What good would it do to find this place again in a world where the greatest religion is science and the logic of the mind? Don't I know this world where emotions and feelings are second-class citizens? Yes, I do. But my teachers have asked me to remind you who you really are. You are more than a human being, much more. Within your heart is a place, a sacred place, where the world can literally be remade through conscious cocreation. If you give me permission, I will show you what has been shown to me."

— Drunvalo Melchizedek

Includes Heart Meditation CD

$25.00 • 144 PP. • Softcover • ISBN 978-1-891824-43-2

All Our Books Are Also Available as eBooks on Amazon, Apple iTunes, Google Play, Barnes & Noble, and Kobo.

⚜ *Light Technology* PUBLISHING *Presents*

TO ORDER PRINT BOOKS
Visit LightTechnology.com, Call 928-526-1345 or 1-800-450-0985,
or Check Amazon.com or Your Favorite Bookstore

BOOKS THROUGH TINA LOUISE SPALDING

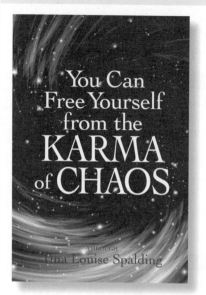

You Can Free Yourself from the Karma of Chaos

We have come here as a group to help you because it is a pivotal time in your planet's evolution. You are seeing monumental changes in your society now. To achieve the shifts that these transfigurations will bring about, you must understand your minds, histories, and human nature as you experience it on the ground, in your hearts, and in your consciousnesses.

Your baggage, judgments, and fears must be released for you to enter this new world, this new time on your planet, with clear and uncontaminated minds. It is our purpose to bring you through this journey so that you will understand, forgive, and walk unencumbered into your new future.

— Ananda

$16.95 • Softcover • 224 PP. • 978-1-62233-057-7

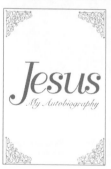

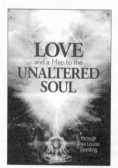

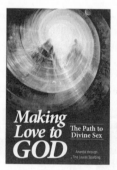

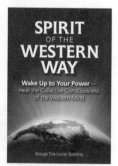

Jesus: My Autobiography
$16.95 • Softcover • 304 PP.
978-1-62233-030-0

**Love and a Map
to the Unaltered Soul**
$16.95 • Softcover • 240 PP.
ISBN 978-1-62233-047-8

**Making Love to God:
The Path to Divine Sex**
$19.95 • Softcover • 416 PP.
978-1-62233-009-6

Great Minds Speak to You
$19.95 • Softcover • 192 PP.
Includes CD
978-1-62233-010-2

**Spirit of the Western Way:
Wake Up to Your Power —
Heal the Collective
Consciousness of the
Western Mind**
$16.95 • Softcover • 176 PP.
978-1-62233-051-5

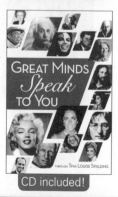

CD included!

All Our Books Are Also Available as eBooks on Amazon, Apple iTunes, Google Play, Barnes & Noble, and Kobo.

TO ORDER PRINT BOOKS
Visit LightTechnology.com, Call 928-526-1345 or 1-800-450-0985,
or Check Amazon.com or Your Favorite Bookstore

BOOKS THROUGH RAE CHANDRAN

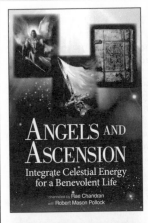

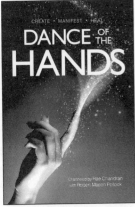

Angels and Ascension
All life's miracles happen with angelic presence. When you aim to communicate with them, you will see that you have an ever-present friend at your shoulder.
$16.95 • Softcover • 176 PP.
ISBN 978-1-62233-048-5

Dance of the Hands
This material is for those who have an interest in bettering themselves or improving their well-being: practitioners, teachers, masters, neophytes, and children.
$16.95 • Softcover • 160 PP.
ISBN 978-1-62233-038-6

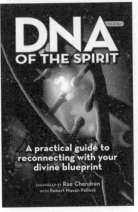

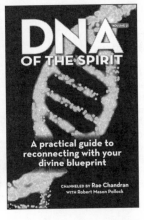

DNA of the Spirit, Volume 1
This is a book about practices you can do and energetic connections you can make to raise your consciousness and activate additional strands of your DNA.
$19.95 • Softcover • 384 PP.
978-1-62233-013-3

DNA of the Spirit, Volume 2
Contained within are methods for experiencing oneness with all, the elements of your physical bodies, and all creation.
$16.95 • Softcover • 192 PP.
978-1-62233-027-0

Partner with Angels
Angels are the Creator's workforce, and here, angels explain how they can help you with all aspects of your life — practical and spiritual. All you need to do is ask.
$16.95 • Softcover • 208 PP.
978-1-62233-034-8

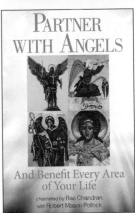

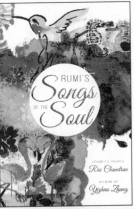

Rumi's Songs of the Soul
Rumi's interest was always to be a bridge between people and God. In this book, Chandran brings Rumi's writings in a newer form suited to the present reality of Earth.
$15.95 • Softcover • 128 PP.
978-1-62233-059-1

COMING SOON
33 Keys to Ascension

All Our Books Are Also Available as eBooks on Amazon, Apple iTunes, Google Play, and Barnes & Noble.

232 ⚜ *Light Technology* PUBLISHING **Presents**

TO ORDER PRINT BOOKS
Visit LightTechnology.com, Call 928-526-1345 or 1-800-450-0985,
or Check Amazon.com or Your Favorite Bookstore

BY TOM T. MOORE

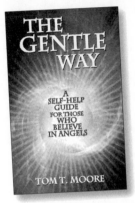

THE GENTLE WAY
A SELF-HELP GUIDE FOR THOSE WHO BELIEVE IN ANGELS

"This book is for people of all faiths and beliefs with the only requirement being a basic belief in angels. It will put you back in touch with your guardian angel or strengthen and expand the connection that you may already have. How can I promise these benefits? Because I have been using these concepts for over ten years and I can report these successes from direct knowledge and experience. But this is a self-help guide, so that means it requires your active participation."   — Tom T. Moore

$14.⁹⁵ • 160 PP. • Softcover • ISBN 978-1-891824-60-9

THE GENTLE WAY II
BENEVOLENT OUTCOMES: THE STORY CONTINUES

You'll be amazed at how easy it is to be in touch with guardian angels and how much assistance you can receive simply by asking. This inspirational self-help book, written for all faiths and beliefs, explains how there is a more benevolent world that we can access and how we can achieve this.

This unique and incredibly simple technique assists you in manifesting your goals easily and effortlessly for the first time. It works quickly, sometimes with immediate results, and no affirmations, written intentions, or changes in behavior are needed. You don't even have to believe in it for it to work!

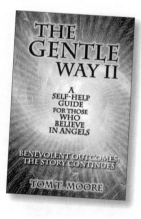

$16.⁹⁵ • 320 PP. • Softcover • ISBN 978-1-891824-80-7

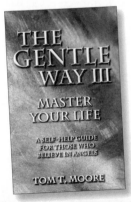

THE GENTLE WAY III
MASTER YOUR LIFE

"Almost three years have passed since *The Gentle Way II* was published. Yet as many success stories as that book contained, I have continued to receive truly unique stories from people all over the world requesting most benevolent outcomes and asking for benevolent prayers for their families, friends, other people, and other beings. It just proves that there are no limits to this modality, which is becoming a gentle movement as people discover how much better their lives are with these simple yet powerful requests."   — Tom T. Moore

$16.⁹⁵ • 352 PP. • Softcover • ISBN 978-1-62233-005-8

All Our Books Are Also Available as eBooks on Amazon, Apple iTunes, Google Play, Barnes & Noble, and Kobo.

§ *Light Technology* PUBLISHING *Presents*   233

TO ORDER PRINT BOOKS
Visit LightTechnology.com, Call 928-526-1345 or 1-800-450-0985,
or Check Amazon.com or Your Favorite Bookstore

SHAMANIC SECRETS SERIES THROUGH ROBERT SHAPIRO

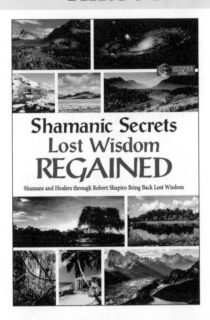

Shamanic Secrets: Lost Wisdom Regained

Due to wars, natural disasters, a shaman not being able to train a successor, and many other reasons, Isis (through Robert) says that 95 percent of the accumulated shamanic wisdom has been lost. Now it is important to regain this wisdom as young people who are able to learn and use these processes are being born now.

Beings who lived as shamans and healers on Earth at various times now speak through Robert Shapiro and bring these lost teachings and techniques to a humanity waking up and discovering it has the talents and abilities to use this wisdom for the benefit of all.

$16.95 • Softcover • 352 PP. • ISBN 978-1-62233-049-2

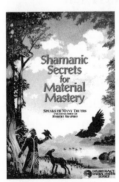

Shamanic Secrets for Material Mastery
Explore the heart and soul connection between humans and Mother Earth. Through that intimacy, miracles of healing and expanded awareness can flourish.
$19.95 • Softcover • 528 PP.
978-1-891824-12-8

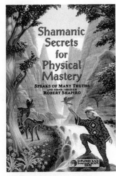

Shamanic Secrets for Physical Mastery
The purpose of this book is to explain the sacred nature of the physical body and some of the magnificent gifts it offers.
$25.00 • Softcover • 608 PP.
978-1-891824-29-6

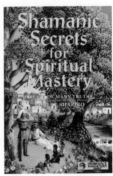

Shamanic Secrets for Spiritual Mastery
Spiritual mastery is the underpinnings of multiple ways of being, understanding, appreciating, and interacting in harmony with your world.
$29.95 • Softcover • 768 PP.
978-1-891824-58-6

All Our Books Are Also Available as eBooks on Amazon, Apple iTunes, Google Play, Barnes & Noble, and Kobo.

234

☦ *Light Technology* PUBLISHING *Presents*

SEDONA JOURNAL OF
Emergence

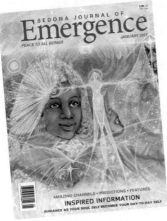

Find Answers to Satisfy Your Heart and Inspire Your Life in the #1 Channeled Magazine for Spiritual Guidance

In the *Sedona Journal of Emergence*, channeled lightbeings explain the process and offer guidance to help you feel and express love and benevolence and to encourage you to make a difference in ensuring Earth's future.

The *Sedona Journal of Emergence* is the one monthly magazine you'll want to keep on hand!

- Mine the annual PREDICTIONS issue for insights on the coming year.
- Discover channeled information and inspired guidance intended to improve your body, mind, and soul.
- Learn how to improve yourself and, by default, help the planet.

DON'T DELAY — SUBSCRIBE TODAY!

SIGN UP ONLINE AT **WWW.SEDONAJOURNAL.COM**,
CALL 1-800-450-0985 OR 1-928-526-1345,

OR EMAIL **SUBSCRIPTIONS@LIGHTTECHNOLOGY.COM.**
(ELECTRONIC SUBSCRIPTIONS AVAILABLE)

☙ *Light Technology* PUBLISHING *Presents*

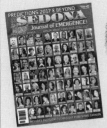

SEDONA JOURNAL OF
Emergence

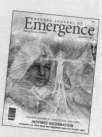

ORDER NOW

to receive SPECTACULAR SAVINGS on your
Sedona Journal subscription!

PRINT SUBSCRIPTIONS

Mailed U.S. Subscriptions

1ˢᵗ CLASS	2ᴺᴰ CLASS
❏ 2yrs $129	❏ 2yrs $79
❏ 1yr $65	❏ 1yr $43

Canada

❏ 2yrs $159	❏ 1yr $83

All prices are in U.S. currency.

All Other Countries

❏ 2yrs $299	❏ 1yr $154

All prices are in U.S. currency.

NOTE: The U.S. Postal Service has changed postal rates, eliminating Canadian and global 2nd class surface and increasing all airmail rates.

Name: _____

Address: _____

City:_____State:_____Zip:_____

Phone:_____Email:_____

Gift Recipient Name: _____

Address: _____

City:_____State:_____Zip:_____

Personalized Gift Card from: _____

METHOD OF PAYMENT (CHECK ONE):

❏ CHECK   ❏ M.O.

❏ VISA   ❏ MASTERCARD   ❏ DISCOVER   ❏ AMEX

CARD NO. _____

EXPIRATION DATE _____

SIGNATURE _____

Subscription includes the annual double-size
PREDICTIONS ISSUE at no extra charge.

ELECTRONIC SUBSCRIPTIONS
with Bonus Content

Get the entire journal plus additional content online by subscription — and get it 2 weeks before it hits newsstands!

❏ 2yrs $55	❏ 1yr $29

All electronic and combo subscriptions *MUST* be purchased online at *www.SedonaJournal.com* to obtain username and password

Get the Best of Both Worlds!
Special Combo Offers!

U.S.A.
Get BOTH Printed AND Electronic Subscriptions

1ˢᵗ CLASS	2ᴺᴰ CLASS
❏ 2yrs $159	❏ 2yrs.........$109
❏ 1yr $81	❏ 1yr $59

Canada
Get an Airmail Printed Subscription Along with an Electronic Subscription for Only

❏ 2yrs $189	❏ 1yr $99

NOTE: The U.S. Postal Service has changed postal rates, eliminating Canadian and global 2nd class surface and increasing all airmail rates.

All Countries
Get an Airmail Printed Subscription Along with an Electronic Subscription for Only

❏ 2yrs $329	❏ 1yr $170

Order online: www.SedonaJournal.com
or call 928-526-1345 or 1-800-450-0985

236 ## 🕯 *Light Technology* PUBLISHING **Presents**

EASY ORDER 24 HOURS A DAY

Order ONLINE!
www.lighttechnology.com

Email:
customersrv@
lighttechnology.net

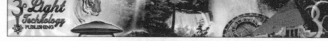

www.LightTechnology.com
We Offer the Best Channeled and Inspired Books of Wisdom.
Use Our Secure Checkout.
In-Depth Information on Books, Including Excerpts and Contents.
Use the Links to Our Other Great Sites. See Below.

Order by Mail
Send To:
Light Technology Publishing
PO Box 3540
Flagstaff, AZ 86003

www.SedonaJournal.com
Read Excerpts of Monthly Channeling and Predictions in Advance.
Use Our Email Links to Contact Us or Send a Submission.
Electronic Subscriptions Available — with or without Print Copies.

Order by Phone
800-450-0985
928-526-1345

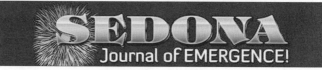

www.BenevolentMagic.com
Learn the techniques of benevolence toward self and benevolence
toward others to create global peace. Download all the techniques
of benevolent magic and living prayer for FREE!

Order by Fax
928-714-1132

Available from your
favorite bookstore or

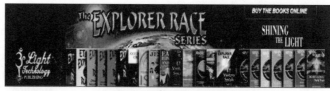

www.ExplorerRace.com
All of humanity constitutes the Explorer Race, volunteers for a grand
and glorious experiment. Discover your purpose, your history, and
your future. Download the first chapter of each book for FREE!

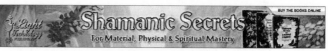

www.ShamanicSecrets.com
What we call shamanism is the natural way of life for beings on other
planets. Learn to be aware of your natural self and your natural talents
and abilities. Download the first chapter of each book for FREE!